A Synopsis of Minor Oral Surgery

A Synopsis of Minor Oral Surgery

George Dimitroulis MDSc (Melb.), FDSRCS (Eng.), FFDRCS (Irel.),
FRACDS (OMS)
Visiting lecturer and clinical demonstrator in
Oral and Maxillofacial Surgery
School of Dental Science,
University of Melbourne

Oral and Maxillofacial Surgeon
Private Practice, Melbourne, Australia

wright

Wright
An imprint of Butterworth-Heinemann
Linacre House, Jordan Hill, Oxford OX2 8DP
225 Wildwood Avenue, Woburn, MA 01801–2041
A division of Reed Educational and Professional Publishing Ltd

R A member of the Reed Elsevier plc group

OXFORD   AUCKLAND   BOSTON
JOHANNESBURG   MELBOURNE   NEW DELHI

First published 1997
Reprinted 1998, 1999, 2000, 2001

British Library Cataloguing in Publication Data
A catalogue record for this book is available from
the British Library

Library of Congress Cataloging in Publication Data
A catalogue record for this book is available from
the Library of Congress

ISBN 0 7236 1094 0

For more information on all Butterworth-Heinemann
publications please visit our website at www.bh.com

Typeset by BC Typesetting, Bristol BS15 5YD
Printed and bound in Great Britain by Biddles Ltd, *www.biddles.co.uk*

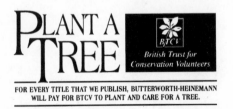

PLANT A TREE

BTCV
*British Trust for
Conservation Volunteers*

FOR EVERY TITLE THAT WE PUBLISH, BUTTERWORTH-HEINEMANN
WILL PAY FOR BTCV TO PLANT AND CARE FOR A TREE.

Contents

Preface

Although dentistry has changed its emphasis remarkably in recent decades from treatment to prevention, minor oral surgery continues to be an integral part of general dental practice. It is therefore important that senior dental students and general dental practitioners appreciate the fundamental principles of minor oral surgery in the light of up-to-date standards of patient care. Instruction in minor oral surgery has for decades been based on a few textbooks that fulfilled the basic requirements of generations of dental students. Although these classic textbooks are still essential for didactic teaching, one must bear in mind that with the constantly changing world of dental and surgical practice, large textbooks can become outdated very quickly.

The aim of this small book is to encompass what is relevant in today's practice of minor oral surgery with the emphasis on total patient care. Every endeavour has been made to present this subject in a logical sequence that is succinct, readable, practical and applicable to everyday clinical practice. I hope that the simplicity and practicality of this book will make oral surgery a more inviting subject for senior dental students to study, and that general dentists will find it a useful reference source for clinical practice. It is envisaged that this book will serve a dual purpose not only as a textbook for the undergraduate dental curriculum but also as a practical guide for contemporary general dental and hospital practice.

George Dimitroulis

1 Setting up practice

Minor oral surgery is the part of dentistry that deals with the diagnosis and surgical treatment of diseases, injuries and defects of the human teeth, jaws, oral cavity and associated structures which, under normal circumstances, can be performed under local anaesthesia in an outpatient setting in most healthy and normal patients.

Before setting up practice in minor oral surgery the clinician must firstly be adequately experienced in the field, and secondly be equipped with various tools of the trade that are essential for the safe practice of minor oral surgery. The aim of this chapter is to present a general guide on how to prepare for minor oral surgery within a general dental office setting.

The waiting room

A successful practice in minor oral surgery is one that is sensitive to the patient's needs, expectations and fears. As well as employing friendly and helpful staff, the clinician must give consideration not only to the functional aspects but also to the aesthetic appeal of the dental office, in particular the waiting room. The key is to create the illusion of a relaxed and warm environment, with 'earth' colour schemes of green, brown and yellow for the walls, carpets, furniture and fixtures, all bathed in yellow lighting. Pictures on the walls should be serene landscapes, and a fish tank is often thought to have a calming effect on most nervous patients. Minor oral surgery is probably the dental procedure that patients fear most, so a calm and relaxed environment goes a long way to easing patients' fears and soothing their nerves prior to surgery.

The operating room

Unlike the general reception area or waiting room, the operating room should convey a sense of complete sterility or cleanliness to the patient, although it should not be too light or bright. Furthermore, every effort should be made to keep the room clear of instruments or complex gadgetry so that the only thing the patient sees on entering the surgery is the dental chair and overhead light. There should ideally be a side-room where the sterilizer and equipment are kept and are wheeled in as soon as the patient is comfortably seated. An ordinary dental chair and light often suffice, but some clinicians may prefer an operating table with powerful lights mounted on an overhead traction, although this would depend on how much minor oral surgery is undertaken in the practice.

Most operations are performed with the clinician standing so there must be plenty of room for the clinician, the assistant and the anaesthetist (if intravenous sedation or inhalation anaesthesia is employed) to move about freely. Music playing softly in the background also helps in setting a relaxed mood for both the staff and the patient. If intravenous sedation or outpatient general anaesthesia is planned then a recovery room adjacent to the operating room is essential, with an exit that avoids the reception area and waiting room.

Surgical instruments

The surgical equipment includes non-disposable instruments and disposable surgical supplies. It is impractical to suggest surgical instruments by brand name so general descriptions of the various instruments are given and it is up to the clinician to choose a particular brand. In minor oral surgery three sets of instruments are used for most operations (Figure 1.1).

Instruments for access and clear surgical field

Access to the surgical site is provided by instruments that not only help to expose the surgical site but also protect the surrounding tissues from inadvertent injury during surgery.

- Mouth prop or gag – placed in the molar teeth to hold the mouth open.
- Cheek retractors.
- Tongue retractors or depressors – expose the lingual alveolus and floor of mouth and keep the tongue protected and well away from the surgical field.
- Flap retractors – expose the surgical site for direct instrumentation.

Maintenance of a clear surgical field essentially involves haemorrhage control by the following methods.

- Suction – aspiration of pooled blood leaked from the surgical wound.
- Fine haemostatic (mosquito) forceps with or without sutures are only used where major vessels are encountered, which is uncommon in minor oral surgery.
- Electrocautery is used for thermal coagulation of bleeding soft tissues. It is particularly useful for tongue and cheek but is not very pleasant for conscious patients.
- Pressure packs (disposable) such as Retec gauze or haemostatic agents such as Gelfoam, Surgicel, bone wax or topical thrombin.

Instruments for manipulation or removal of surgical specimen

The specimen may be soft tissue, bone or teeth.

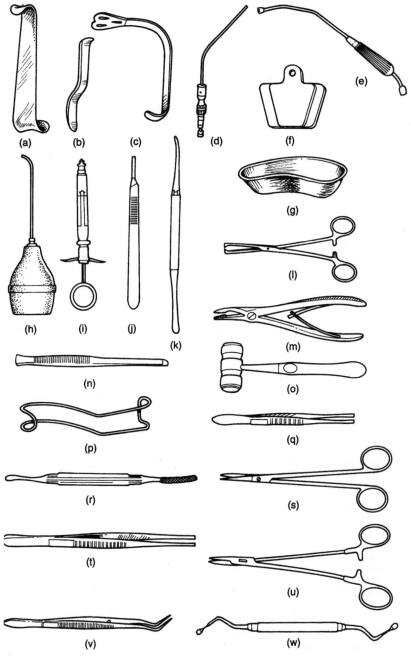

Figure 1.1 Basic instrument tray: a, Kilner cheek retractor; b, Minnesota retractor; c, tongue depressor/retractor; d, fine-tip surgical suction; e, Yankeur suction; f, rubber mouth prop; g, kidney dish; h, irrigation bulb and tip; i, aspirating local anaesthetic syringe; j, scalpel handle; k, periosteal elevator; l, Allis tissue forceps; m, bone-cutting rongeur; n, chisel; o, mallet; p, wire cheek retractor; q, fragment forceps; r, bone file; s, suture scissors; t, rat-toothed tissue forceps; u, needle holder; v, curved pick-up forceps; w, bi-angled curette.

SOFT TISSUE SURGERY

Instruments used to establish a surgical pathway to the surgical specimen are:

- Scalpel – scalpel handle with disposable blade (usually no. 15 blade in minor oral surgery). The scalpel handle must be gripped like a pen and the incision made towards the operator. Incisions should be made down to bone in one clean sweep; avoid going over the same incision more than once.
- Periosteal elevator – used to raise or bluntly dissect a mucoperiosteal flap off the bone.
- Dissection scissors – come in various sizes and patterns. Confined mainly to soft tissue surgery.

BONE SURGERY

- Chisel and mallet.
- Osteotome – bevelled on both sides, the osteotome is often used to split bone rather than being used like a chisel to whittle it away.
- Bone forceps such as the rongeur are used to trim bony projections by grasping and slicing using sharp beaks.
- Bone file – used manually to smooth over sharp bony projections.
- Powered handpiece and burr – an essential tool in minor oral surgery. The handpiece must have high torque strength with the exhaust (if air-powered) facing away from the surgical site. Surgical burrs are often made of stainless steel or tungsten carbide and have a long shank, and are either round (size 6 to 8) or fissured (usually size 701 or 702). Sometimes fast-cutting jet burrs or large acrylic burrs for grinding may be used. Coolant sterile irrigation fluid must always be used with powered handpieces to avoid overheating the bone.

DENTAL EXTRACTIONS

- Dental forceps – see below.
- Dental elevators – see below.
- Sectioning teeth – osteotome or powered handpiece and burr (see above).

Instruments for wound toilet and repair

- Tissue or fragment forceps – for picking out loose tissue debris within the wound.
- Curette – used in a scraping or scooping fashion to clear up fragments of soft tissue adherent to bony cavities.
- Irrigation syringe – filled with sterile isotonic irrigation fluid such as saline to clean out microscopic debris from wound.
- Suture set – used to repair the wound through primary closure of the surgical defect. Comprises the following:
    needle holder
    toothed tissue forceps – for picking up and stabilizing the tissue to be

sutured
suture scissors
sutures – see below.

Dental forceps

In the practice of minor oral surgery, dental forceps are essential and are among the most commonly used surgical instruments. Dental forceps are designed in a large number of patterns, styles and configurations which adapt to the different teeth and variety of techniques used to extract teeth (Figure 1.2).

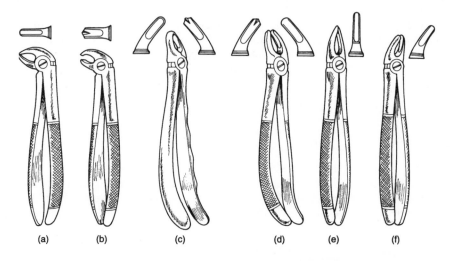

(a)	(b)	(c)	(d)	(e)	(f)

Figure 1.2 Dental forceps: a, lower universal forceps; b, lower anatomical (hawk's-bill) forceps; c, upper right anatomical forceps; d, upper left anatomical forceps; e, upper straight forceps; f, upper curved (or universal) forceps.

Basic components

HANDLE

The handle is serrated to allow a firm grip and prevent slippage. The length is designed to allow the operator to deliver sufficient pressure and leverage to extract the tooth from its bony socket.

HINGE

As the connection between the handle and the beaks, the hinge has an important function in transferring and concentrating the force applied from the handle to the beaks.

BEAKS

The beaks comprise the working end of the instrument, which is designed to adapt to the root rather than the crown of the tooth. The beaks constitute the greatest source of variation among forceps depending on the root configuration of each tooth, so that the width, tip and angulation of the beaks are designed for close adaptation to the tooth parallel to its long axis to permit the most mechanically efficient means for extraction.

International differences

Dental forceps designs have evolved differently in the British Commonwealth countries and North America. The different designs and patterns are a reflection of the different techniques of patient positioning with respect to the clinician and the different methods of handling the forceps. The British forceps technique provides greater leverage, although it may be more likely to result in crown fracture because of the greater forces generated compared with the American forceps.

Use of dental forceps

The clinical use of dental forceps is discussed in Chapter 4.

Dental elevators

Dental elevators are the other most commonly used surgical instruments in minor oral surgery (Figure 1.3). These instruments are particularly useful in surgical extractions (see Chapter 5).

Basic components

HANDLE

The larger the handle, the greater is the force that can be applied.

SHANK

The shank is the connection that transmits the force from the handle to the blade.

BLADE

The blade is the working tip of the instrument that contacts the tooth and bone. The working side of the blade (the side facing the tooth to be extracted) is usually flat or concave.

Different designs

The largest variation in the type and design of an elevator is in the shape and size of the blade. The elevators are either straight or curved depending

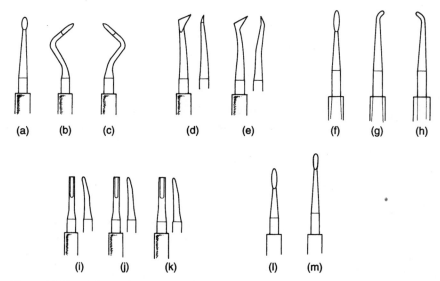

Figure 1.3 Dental elevators: a, clinic straight exolever; b, clinic left exolever; c, clinic right exolever; d, Cryer's elevator 30 (left); e, Cryer's elevator 31 (right); f, Warwick-James straight; g, Warwick-James left; h, Warwick-James right; i, Coupland bone chisel 1; j, Coupland bone chisel 2; k, Coupland bone chisel 3; l, apical elevator E80; m, apical elevator E301.

on the direction of the blade tip relative to the shank. Examples of *straight elevators* are straight Warwick-James, Coupland 1, 2 and 3, and Cogswell A. Examples of *curved elevators* are left and right Warwick-James, left and right Cryer's, and Cogswell B.

Principles of use

Using a point of purchase or fulcrum (e.g. alveolar crestal bone), a rotatory motion is used to lever and luxate the tooth or root fragment from its socket.

Clinical applications

The clinical applications (see also Chapter 5) are:

- To luxate teeth – to loosen teeth from the surrounding bone in order to facilitate forceps extraction.
- To expand the bone socket for easier application of forceps and greater mobility of tooth.
- To remove broken or surgically sectioned dental fragments from their bony crypt or socket.

Sutures

Suturing is a technique that every dentist should be familiar with.

Types of suture

Sutures may be absorbable or non-absorbable.

ABSORBABLE SUTURES

Organic
The most common example of an organic absorbable suture is catgut made of twisted collagen from the intestines of sheep or cattle. *Plain catgut* is absorbed unpredictably by phagocytosis and the ensuing inflammatory reaction results in early loss of tensile strength (after a few days). *Chromic catgut* is coated with a chromic solution which helps to prolong the absorption period of the suture.

Synthetic
Synthetic sutures consist of braided fibres of polyglycolic acid (Dexon), polyglactin (Vicryl) and polydioxanone (PDS) which are stronger than catgut, with better handling, less tissue reaction and a longer half-life (loss of 50% tensile strength in 2 weeks).

NON-ABSORBABLE SUTURES

Organic
Silk is the most common example but has largely been superseded by synthetic materials, since its braided nature attracts infection by capillary action. Other organic sutures such as cotton and linen are rarely used.

Synthetic
Examples such as Prolene, nylon and Surgilon may be braided or monofilament; the latter is relatively inert with little tissue reaction. Capillary action in the braided sutures may be reduced by a coating of polytetrafluoroethylene which renders them smooth. Complications of non-absorbable sutures include sinus formation, especially where the surgical wound toilet is poor.

Types of needle

Most sutures come fused to a needle in pre-sterilized packaging. Suture needles differ according to the shape of their cross-section and their length (Figure 1.4).

- **Cross-section** – There are generally two types:
   Cutting needles have a triangular cross-section with the apex of the triangle at the concavity of the needle. Reverse cutting needles have the apex on the convexity and are less traumatic
   Taper-point needles are round or oval in cross-section and are rarely used in minor oral surgery.
- **Length** – Again, there are two types:
   Straight needles – only used where tissues are easily accessible and therefore have no use in minor oral surgery

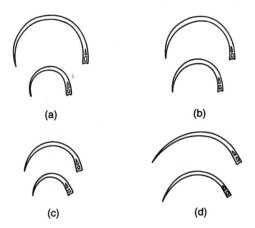

Figure 1.4 Suture needles: a, half-circle round body needles; b, half-circle tapered (cutting) needles; c, 3/8 round body needles; d, 3/8 tapered (cutting) needles.

Curved needles – the most commonly used are the 3/8 needles, although deeper tissues with more restricted access may require half-circle needles.

Size of sutures

The gauge or the calibre of suture is expressed in numbers whereby the smallest sutures used for microsurgical work are in the 10/0, 9/0 and 8/0 categories, going up in size to 3/0, 2/0 and 1/0 being the largest, although in other surgical specialties there are larger sutures such as 0/0, etc. In minor oral surgery practice the 3/0 is most commonly used, although the smaller 4/0 may sometimes be used for delicate areas such as the floor of the mouth and the labial mucosa.

Tying sutures

The technique of tying sutures should be demonstrated by an experienced clinician and then practised on a rubber dam before it is attempted on a patient.

METHOD

There are two methods of tying sutures:

- Instrument tying – the knot is established by passing the suture once (square knot) or twice (surgeon's knot) around the tip of the needle holder. The knot is tightened and then locked by passing the suture around the needle holder in the opposite direction (Figure 1.5).
- Hand tying is rarely used in minor oral surgery practice.

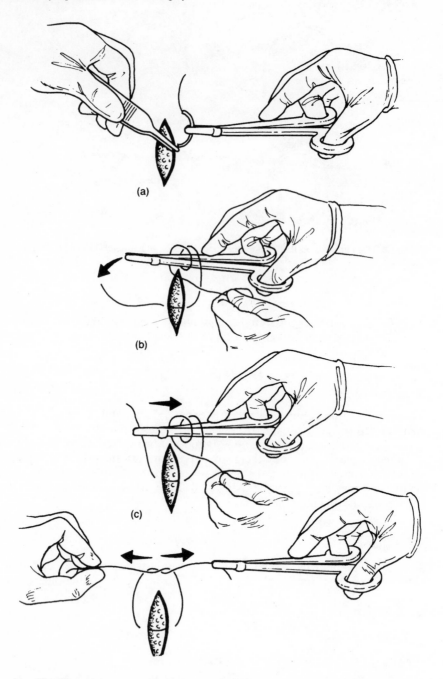

Figure 1.5 Instrument suturing technique: a, tissue forceps are used to lift and stabilize the wound margin to allow passage of suture; b, one or two throws of the suture are made around the needle holder; c, the free end of the suture is grasped with the needle holder and passed through the loops; d, with the suture needle held in one hand and the needle holder in the other, the knot is completed as the two ends are drawn apart.

SUTURING PATTERNS

In minor oral surgery the most common pattern is the simple interrupted suture followed by the horizontal mattress suture which is used to hold together soft tissues over a tooth extraction socket. Other patterns which are more common on the skin are the continuous overhand (baseball) stitch and the continuous subcuticular sutures (Figure 1.6).

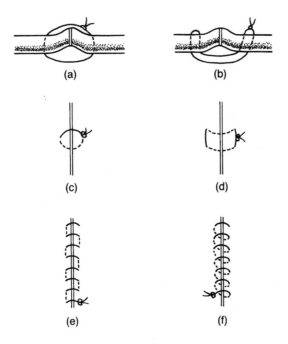

(a)   (b)

(c)   (d)

(e)   (f)

Figure 1.6 Common suture patterns: a, cross-sectional view of a simple interrupted suture – note the slight eversion of the wound margins and the knot placed to one side; b, cross-sectional view of a horizontal mattress suture; c, simple interrupted suture; d, horizontal mattress suture; e, continuous cross stitch; f, continuous overhand (baseball) stitch.

Suture technique

In the practice of minor oral surgery, the following hints should be borne in mind when suturing.

1. Normally suture from free to fixed tissues, taking a bite of approximately 3 mm on each side of the wound margin. In some situations such as palate to buccal mucosa, suturing from fixed to free tissues may be required.
2. Avoid too much tension when closing wounds.
3. Leave the sutured wound edges slightly everted in apposition.
4. Preferably use resorbable sutures, particularly in areas of the oral cavity where access is limited or poor, e.g. third molar extraction sites.

5. Make the closure over deeper supporting tissue; for example, it is better for wound margins to rest on bone rather than over a cystic cavity where there is a high incidence of wound breakdown.
6. Non-resorbable sutures used in the oral cavity are best removed in 7 days unless they are used to hold a pack in place in which case they may remain longer.

Remember: in most cases, the type of suture used becomes a matter of personal preference.

Cross-infection in dental practice

Aseptic technique is prudent for all surgical procedures where the risk of cross-infection is especially significant, such as minor oral surgery.

Modes of transmission

1. Splatter (eyes).
2. Aerosol – air turbine surgical handpiece.
3. Direct contact with saliva or blood – e.g. needle-stick injury.
4. Indirect contact – poorly cleaned surgical instruments.

Infection control in clinical practice

PATIENT SCREENING

Identify high-risk groups for hepatitis and human immunodeficiency virus (HIV) infection.

BARRIER METHODS

Personal protection requires not only adequate hand-washing but also the wearing of gloves, mask, gown, glasses and cap.

ASEPTIC TECHNIQUE

A 'no touch' policy is facilitated by proper office design such as elbow taps for hand-washing, foot controls for chair adjustment and sterile detachable handles for overhead lights.

INSTRUMENT STERILIZATION

Destruction of all contaminating life forms including viruses and spores is most effectively achieved with an autoclave (see below), an essential piece of equipment for all clinical practices. For heat-sensitive instruments, a 2% glutaraldehyde solution is best (see below).

SURFACE DISINFECTION

Work benches, instrument trays and dental chairs are best disinfected with an iodoform spray (see below).

DISPOSAL OF SHARPS AND WASTE

Sharps and waste should be carefully handled, ensuring safety at all times so that accidental pricks and spillage of suctioned fluids and blood do not occur.

Ethical considerations in minor oral surgery

The risk of a dentist acquiring a transmissible disease through the practice of minor oral surgery is low, presuming the dentist exercises sound basic clinical hygiene at all times. Dentists, like other health professionals, have a professional and human obligation to treat and care for all patients including those with hepatitis and HIV infections. Denying patients access to treatment will only lead to their frustration and, in many cases, to probable future concealment of their infection from other practitioners.

Heat sterilization of instruments

Surgical instruments may be sterilized in one of three ways.

AUTOCLAVE

The autoclave is probably the most commonly used sterilization technique available today. It must be regularly monitored and well maintained. Although expensive, it is safe and reliable, but can corrode some instruments. Latent heat of water, 134 °C for 4 minutes or 121 °C for 15 minutes.

DRY HEAT

Hot air ovens are much cheaper to purchase and maintain than autoclaves but their cycles, which may be interrupted, are much longer: 60 minutes at 160 °C or 30 minutes at 180 °C.

CHEMICLAVE

A mixture of ethyl alcohol, formaldehyde, isopropyl alcohol, acetone and ketone is heated to 132 °C for 20 minutes. It is expensive to run but does not corrode instruments, although a scavenger system is required to contain the noxious vapours released.

Chemical disinfection

Used to treat heat-sensitive equipment, furniture and fixtures, chemical disinfection may be accomplished with the following solutions.

GLUTARALDEHYDE

A 2% glutaraldehyde solution has a broad antimicrobial spectrum which is effective within 30 minutes. It is sporicidal in 7–10 hours at room temperature.

- **Advantages:**
  non-corrosive to stainless steel
  penetrates blood, pus and organic debris
  has a prolonged activated shelf-life.
- **Disadvantages:**
  allergenic to skin and mucous membrane.

IODOFORM

Iodoform is highly effective and recommended as a hard surface disinfectant.

- **Advantages:**
  residual biocidal action on hard surfaces continues for some time after the surface is dry.
- **Disadvantages:**
  may discolour light-coloured surfaces with repeated use
  corrosive to some metals.

OTHER CHEMICAL DISINFECTANTS

Alcohol, phenolic compounds, chlorines and quaternary ammonium compounds are less effective and should be used with caution.

Further reading

Kirk RM (1989) *Basic Surgical Techniques*. 3rd edn. Edinburgh: Churchill Livingstone.

Moore JR, Gillbe GV (1991) *Principles of Oral Surgery*. 4th edn, pp 60–74. Manchester University Press.

Samaranayake LP, Scheutz F, Cottone JA (1990) *Infection Control for the Dental Team*. Copenhagen: Munksgaard.

Scully C, Cawson RA, Griffiths M (1990) *Occupational Hazards to Dental Staff*. London: British Dental Journal Publishing.

Seward M (ed.) *Into Dental Practice*. London: British Dental Journal Publishing.

2 Patient preparation

Although surgical technique is a skill that can only be mastered through clinical experience, it should be emphasized that perioperative care of the patient is what distinguishes a health professional from a skilled technician. Prior to undertaking minor oral surgery, the clinician must be certain that the planned surgical procedure will adequately address the patient's presenting complaints. Furthermore, the onus is on the clinician to determine whether the patient is physically and mentally fit enough to undergo a minor surgical procedure under local anaesthesia in an outpatient setting such as a private dental office. The purpose of this chapter is to outline the essential steps required to prepare a patient for minor oral surgery.

Terminology

Symptom – a subjective problem that a patient describes, such as pain.
Sign – an abnormal presentation that is readily detectable by the clinician, such as a swelling.

Getting to the problem

To prepare the patient for minor oral surgery, the clinician must follow three important steps that will enable the most appropriate course of action to be formulated.

1. History:
   chief presenting complaint
   history of presenting complaint
   medical history
   social history.
2. Examination:
   extraoral examination
   intraoral examination
   investigations.
3. Decision:
   diagnosis
   treatment planning.

History

The first encounter with a patient presenting for minor oral surgery must establish a working diagnosis which always begins with a verbal history from the patient. The clinician must cultivate the essential art of listening and gently directing the conversation so that the patient keeps to the problem in question and does not introduce irrelevant issues.

CHIEF PRESENTING COMPLAINT

The clinician must determine what is the patient's main concern. The most common presenting complaint is pain. Since pain is a subjective phenomenon, a detailed history of the site, nature, duration and extent of pain is essential in order to determine the cause and pathology. Other presenting problems may include:

- Swelling.
- Tooth mobility.
- Discharge and foul taste.
- Asymptomatic oral pathology picked up on routine oral examination.
- Asymptomatic retained roots or impacted teeth picked up on routine radiological screening.

It is important to realize that the chief presenting complaint is pivotal to the overall management of the patient.

HISTORY OF THE PRESENTING COMPLAINT

Background information about the presenting complaint will often provide the clinician with a clearer understanding of the cause and nature of the condition. Questions that may be important in building up a background picture of the patient's presenting condition may include:

- When the problem was first noticed by the patient.
- Possible cause of the problem, e.g. biting into something hard and hearing a crack in the tooth with a sudden shooting pain.
- The natural course of the problem, e.g. continuously present, or comes and goes with a certain frequency.
- Any treatment sought in the past and the outcome, e.g. a course of antibiotics helped reduce the pain and swelling.

MEDICAL HISTORY

In an outpatient dental setting it is impractical for the clinician to delve into a detailed medical and systems history for all patients (see Chapter 17). Instead, a brief but adequate screening medical history is usually sufficient to pick out patients who require more investigation (Figure 2.1). One commonly used example of a screening medical history is as follows:

1. Allergies – particularly to commonly used antibiotics and analgesics.
2. Medication – check specifically for steroids, insulin and anticoagulant therapy.

U.R. No.	ROYAL DENTAL HOSPITAL

U.R. No.
Mr.
SURNAME Mrs.
Miss.
Ms.
GIVEN NAMES
DATE OF BIRTH

**ROYAL DENTAL HOSPITAL
OF MELBOURNE**

QUESTIONS CONCERNING GENERAL HEALTH

TICK YOUR ANSWER IN THE SQUARE — YES — NO

Have you ever had – heart trouble? ☐ ☐
high blood pressure? ☐ ☐
a stroke? ☐ ☐

chest trouble? ☐ ☐
asthma? ☐ ☐

arthritis? ☐ ☐
rheumatism? ☐ ☐

rheumatic fever? ☐ ☐
hepatitis? ☐ ☐
diabetes? ☐ ☐
fits or epilepsy? ☐ ☐
allergies? ☐ ☐

Have you visited a MEDICAL DOCTOR in the last 3 months? ☐ ☐

Have you taken any tablets or medicine in the last month? ☐ ☐

Have you EVER had any serious illness? ☐ ☐

Have you had a general anaesthetic or an operation of any kind? ☐ ☐

Have you had bleeding needing special treatment? ☐ ☐

Does Penicillin or any other medicine make you sick or upset you? ☐ ☐

Has dental treatment ever made you sick? ☐ ☐

Have you ever used addictive drugs? ☐ ☐

Are you pregnant? ☐ ☐

If you are in a group which is susceptible to "A.I.D.S.", PLEASE INFORM YOUR DENTAL OFFICER.
This will NOT prevent you receiving treatment.
The "AT RISK" groups are:–
  a) Males who have engaged in homosexual activity during the previous five years.
  b) Males or females who take drugs by injection into veins.
  c) Males or females who are suffering from a combination of night sweats, unexplained fever, weight loss and persistent swollen glands.
  d) Recipients of blood or blood products e.g. blood transfusion.
  e) Sexual partners of any of the above.

Sign Here: _____   Date: _____

Figure 2.1 Medical history questionnaire. Note the simplicity of the wording and presentation which should make it easy for all literate patients to understand and complete.

3. Major illnesses – especially rheumatic fever, heart valve disorders, history of myocardial infarct or strokes (including transient ischaemic attacks), diabetes mellitus, fits or epilepsy, asthma, thyroid dysfunction, chronic renal failure and bleeding disorders.
4. Previous operations – in particular, open heart surgery, organ transplant surgery or ablative cancer surgery. The patient should also be asked about any unusual reactions to general anaesthesia.

Note: the medical history above specifically targets medical conditions that have a direct influence on the way the minor oral surgery will be carried out. A more detailed appraisal of the management of the medically compromised patient is given in Chapter 15.

SOCIAL HISTORY

The social history should specifically include the patient's social habits and practices rather than be simply a family portrait. Although it may be of some embarrassment to patients, it is important (preferably in a subtle and diplomatic way) to extract the following information:

● Smoking history.
● Alcohol intake.
● Pregnancy status.
● History of injecting drug abuse.
● Sexual practices – male homosexuals or bisexuals.

The most significant aspect of the social history is to determine the patient's risk status for hepatitis B or HIV. This is discussed further in Chapter 15.

Examination

In clinical practice, examination of the patient involves four routine procedures.

1. Inspection. At the start of every examination you must begin by looking at the patient as a whole before looking at the region in question for signs that may provide clues for a diagnosis.
2. Palpation. Next, use your fingertips to feel for tender spots, lumps, fluctuant swellings and mobile teeth.
3. Percussion. In minor oral surgery, percussion or tapping is mainly confined to tapping teeth to elicit symptoms of pain or tenderness, unlike in medicine where finger percussion is used to establish the resonance quality and degree of consolidation of a particular organ (lung fields) or body cavity (abdomen).
4. Auscultation. Although checking for particular sounds within the body using a stethoscope is particularly useful in medicine, auscultation in minor oral surgery has little relevance apart from assessing sounds emanating from the temporomandibular joints.

EXTRAORAL EXAMINATION

Inspection

In minor oral surgery, observation is mainly confined to the head and neck area. However, the initial assessment of the patient must always begin with the general appearance of the patient. The following routine of extraoral inspection may be useful:

- General appearance: does the patient look ill, febrile, fatigued (been up all night with pain), weak, distressed, thin or grossly obese?
- Facial appearance: any obvious facial asymmetry or gross facial swelling? Skin colour and texture – is a rash present?
- Trismus: limited degree of mouth opening.

Palpation

- Neck lumps, such as tender submandibular lymph nodes.
- Gross facial swelling: does it feel hot or fluctuant to indicate an abscess?
- Skin colour and texture: is the bright red colour firm and tender to palpation, indicating a cellulitis?

INTRAORAL EXAMINATION

Strong light is essential. Gentle use of dental mirror and cheek retractors is conducive to good rapport with the patient.

Inspection

It is always best to inspect the teeth last as it is often too easy to overlook other pathology within the oral cavity when the teeth are commonly the site of most of the surgical pathology within the mouth.

- Tongue: check size, degree of mobility, colour and texture.
- Oral mucosa: begin with the palate, cheeks, labial mucosa and floor of mouth, checking for any changes in colour, texture, ulcers, lumps and so on.
- Alveolar ridges and gingivae: assess colour, texture, degree of recession (gingivae), ulcers and lumps.
- Teeth: check for number and position of teeth, large restorations, crowns, gross carious lesions, cracked or missing cusps, exposed dentine, cementum or pulps.

Palpation

- Soft tissues: check for tenderness, consistency of lumps, and fluctuance of any swelling that may be present.
- Teeth: check mobility and use a dental probe to assess defective restoration margins, interproximal carious lesions and periodontal pocketing, or for pus discharge under an inflamed operculum surrounding a partly erupted tooth.

Percussion
A tooth may be tapped with the handle of a dental mirror to elicit pain due to apical periodontitis, usually in a non-vital tooth.

INVESTIGATIONS

Investigations provide additional information that cannot be obtained by history and physical examination. The clinician must be acutely aware of the expense involved and should balance this with the value of the information being sought in dictating treatment strategies. In minor oral surgery practice, the most commonly used investigations are as follows:

Periapical dental radiographs
Periapical radiography is essential when there is a history of difficult extractions or where surgical exodontia is planned (see Chapter 5).

Orthopantomograph
An orthopantomograph (Figure 2.2) is an excellent general screening radiograph of the teeth and jaws, but consideration of cost and irradiation to the patient should dictate a sensible approach to its use.

Pulp testing
Pulp testing is sometimes useful to assess vitality of teeth in cases where the signs and symptoms are equivocal.

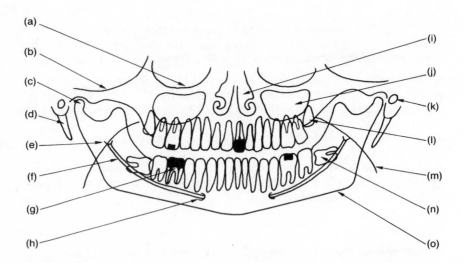

Figure 2.2 Schematic diagram of orthopantomogram: a, orbital floor; b, zygomatic arch; c, condylar process; d, styloid process; e, mandibular foramen and lingula; f, inferior dental canal; g, crowned and root-treated molar; h, mental foramen; i, nasal cavity; j, maxillary sinus; k, internal acoustic meatus; l, impacted upper third molar; m, outline of soft palate; n, impacted lower third molar; o, mandibular angle.

Haematologic tests
Haematological tests are not commonly used in an outpatient setting unless the patient has a bleeding diathesis (see Chapter 15).

Note: investigations play a greater role within a hospital environment and this is discussed in greater detail in Chapter 17.

Decision

Based on the information obtained through the history and examination, the clinician must deduce a working summary of the patient's problems (diagnosis) and decide on the best course of action (treatment plan).

DIAGNOSIS

A diagnosis is a clinical summary of the patient's presenting condition. It should accurately reflect the underlying pathology and the clinical signs and symptoms of disease. In this way, a diagnosis will not only permit communication between clinicians, but will also help in determining the most appropriate course of action.

TREATMENT PLANNING

An accurate diagnosis is the key to planning the most appropriate course of action. The treatment selected should address the patient's chief presenting complaint as well as eliminate all contributing factors that serve to maintain or nurture the disease process. For example, drainage of a dental abscess must always be followed by the elimination of the source of the infection, such as extraction of a non-vital tooth that cannot be restored.

Where multiple problems are present, treatment priority should be given to conditions that are of greatest concern to the patient, e.g. extraction of a painful tooth before excision of a mucocele.

Patient consent

Once all the clinical data are gathered, a working diagnosis established and a treatment plan formulated, the next step is to obtain the consent of the patient prior to embarking on treatment. A patient who has agreed to a proposed surgical plan is in fact consenting to undergo treatment. The basis for consent is a well-informed patient who ultimately has the final say on whether to proceed with treatment.

Patient rights

Unlike the 'old days', clinicians are under scrutiny by an increasingly educated community, encouraged by the expanding legal profession and enterprising mass media keen to sell stories that hit at the heart of human suffering. As a result, clinicians are becoming more attuned to the rights of their patients than ever before – so much so, that there is a trend towards advising patients of their treatment options rather than dictating treatment protocol.

Informing the patient

When informing the patient about the proposed treatment, simple language must be used for the sake of clarity and understanding. Ultimately, the patient should be able to comprehend fully the nature of the procedure and the anticipated outcome. During the consultation the clinician should be prepared to pause at intervals, and allow the patient a chance to digest the information and ask questions. It is impossible to gauge how much the patient has understood if the conversation remains totally one-sided.

Treatment options

It must be stressed that patients should always be informed of their options and should never be led to believe that there are no alternatives. Therefore the option of no treatment and its consequences must always be discussed so that the patient can make an informed and well-balanced decision.

Written or verbal consent?

Where patients' levels of consciousness are to be impaired by sedation or general anaesthesia, then a written consent signed by both the patient and the clinician, preferably in the presence of a witness who also signs, is mandatory prior to surgery. If the surgical procedure is undertaken under local anaesthesia alone, verbal consent by the patient is usually sufficient. In many parts of the USA, however, patients are often required to give written consent for *all* treatment, even when the treatment is under local anaesthesia alone.

Criteria for written consent

The consent form must have the patient's full name, a description of the proposed operation, the date, the patient's full signature, the full signature of a witness other than the surgeon, and the signature of the clinician who has discussed the planned procedure with the patient (Figure 2.3).

Consent for minors and mentality handicapped patients

Consent for these patients must be sought from a parent or legal guardian prior to treatment.

CONSENT TO OPERATIVE TREATMENT
AND ADMINISTRATION OF ANAESTHETIC

I, ... *John Barry Smithson* .... hereby consent to the

following operation(s) .... *Surgical removal of 4 wisdom teeth* ....

being performed on .... *Myself* ....

The nature and effect of the above operation has been explained

to me by Dr .... *George Dimitroulis* ....

I also consent to such further treatment as may be found necessary
to preserve my life and health during the course of the operation(s)
stated above. I also consent to the administration of such anaesthetics
as may be considered necessary by the anaesthetist.

I accept all risks involved in these procedures and agree to be transferred
to another institution if the need arises for further care that is not
available in this institution.

Dated this .... *14th* .... day of .... *May* .... 19 *96* ....

Signed .... Relationship to patient .... *Self* ....

Signature of witness .... Signature of doctor/dentist ....

Figure 2.3 Consent form. A written consent form should be completed by every patient who is to undergo an operative procedure that will involve impaired conscious levels, i.e. sedation and general anaesthesia.

Further reading

Layton S, Korsen J (1994) Informed consent in oral and maxillofacial surgery: a study of the value of written warnings. *Br J Oral Maxillofac Surg*, **32**, 34–36.

Porter SR, Scully C (1991) *Radiographic Interpretation of Orofacial Disease*. Oxford: Oxford Medical.

Scully C (1989) *Patient Care – A Dental Surgeon's Guide*. London: British Dental Journal.

Turner R, Blackwood R (1990) *Lecture Notes on History Taking and Examination*. Oxford: Blackwell.

Wagner JD, Moore DL (1991) Preoperative laboratory testing for the oral and maxillofacial surgery patient. *J Oral Maxillofac Surg*, **49**, 177–182.

3 Anaesthesia

For maximum patient comfort and cooperation, anaesthesia has become an inseparable part of surgery, without which current surgical advancements could not have been achieved. In minor oral surgery, local anaesthesia is the mainstay in patient management, although patients also have the option of general anaesthesia or simply local anaesthesia supplemented with sedation for greater patient convenience.

Terminology

Anaesthesia – absence of sensory input resulting either from injury to sensory nerve pathways, or pharmacologically as a deliberate attempt to eliminate the perception of noxious stimuli (i.e. pain) arising from surgical procedures.

Local anaesthesia

In dentistry, local anaesthetic solutions are conveniently packaged in disposable, single-use 2 ml glass cartridges that are inserted into reuseable dental syringes with a screw attachment for disposable needles. Local anaesthesia forms an indispensable part of the minor oral surgery armamentarium.

- **Advantages:**
    safe, efficient and predictably effective in almost all patients
    inexpensive
    easy to administer
    no monitoring equipment required in healthy patients
    patient remains fully conscious with an intact gag reflex
    outpatient procedure (convenient for patients)
    no preoperative fasting required
    immediate discharge without the need for a recovery period or an escort.
- **Limitations:**
    unsuitable for uncooperative patients (e.g. small children), patients who are afraid of needles, and anxious or very nervous patients
    only suitable for short procedures (less than 30 minutes duration)
    often difficult to anaesthetize inflamed tissues adequately.

Local anaesthetic solutions

CONTENTS

Local anaesthetic solutions consists of:

  local anaesthetic base
  hydrochloride salts for solubility and stability
  vasoconstrictors – adrenaline or felypressin (Octapressin)
  buffering agents
  preservatives – parabens (benzoic acid derivatives).

PHARMACOLOGY

Local anaesthetic agents are weak alkalis and are composed of three parts:

- Amino group – hydrophilic and ionizable.
- Aromatic ring – lipophilic and non-ionizable.
- Amide link – connects the amino group to the aromatic ring.

They are converted in liver or plasma to a water-soluble metabolite and excreted in urine.

MECHANISM OF ACTION

The local anaesthetic agent reversibly blocks impulse conduction along the nerve axon by binding to sodium channels, thus blocking sodium influx through the membrane. The drug is absorbed into neural tissues via simple diffusion in the non-ionized form. Once in the cell the drug is ionized and activated by the intracellular acidic environment. In the acidic environment of inflamed tissues, the drug becomes ionized and cannot diffuse into the neural cell.

TYPES OF LOCAL ANAESTHETIC SOLUTIONS

The three most commonly used local anaesthetic solutions in minor oral surgery are lignocaine, prilocaine and bupivacaine.

Lignocaine (Xylocaine)
First synthesized in 1943, lignocaine has become the most popular of all local anaesthetic solutions. It provides excellent anaesthesia of about 1.5 hours duration. The drug is available as a 2% solution (20 mg/ml) in a 2 ml cartridge (40 mg) plain or with 1:80 000 adrenaline. The maximum safe limit is 200 mg (10 ml of 2% plain solution) or 500 mg (25 ml of 2% solution with 1:80 000 adrenaline).

Prilocaine (Citanest)
Prilocaine is used as an alternative to lignocaine with adrenaline in patients with a history of hypertension, ischaemic heart disease and hyperthyroidism.

It has a slower onset than lignocaine with a shorter half-life. Prilocaine is 40% less toxic than lignocaine, although it may cause methaemoglobinaemia in high doses. It is available as a 4% solution (40 mg/ml) in a 2 ml cartridge (80 mg) plain or with felypressin (Octapressin). The maximum safe limit is 400 mg (10 ml of 4% plain solution).

Bupivacaine (Marcain)

Bupivacaine is long-acting (8–10 hours), because it is highly tissue-bound. It is excellent for immediate postoperative pain control. The onset of action is slow (30 minutes); adrenaline speeds up onset but has little effect on the duration of action. Bupivacaine is available in strengths of 0.2%, 0.5% and 0.75% plain, 0.25% with 1: 400 000 adrenaline and 0.5% with 1: 200 000 adrenaline.

VASOCONSTRICTORS

Vasoconstrictors retard the removal of the local anaesthetic agent from the injection site, thereby increasing the duration of action of the agent, decreasing the blood levels and therefore lowering the toxicity.

Adrenaline

Adrenaline is a natural catecholamine which constricts small arteries in skin and mucosa. Although it also increases cardiac work and output, it does not alter mean arterial blood pressure.

Felypressin (Octapressin)

A synthetic analogue of the naturally occurring vasopressin, felypressin is less effective in haemorrhage control since it only constricts venous outflow.

Contraindications

- Adrenaline – avoid where there is a history of hypertension, hyperthyroidism, ischaemic heart disease or insulin dependent diabetes mellitus, or when halothane is being used.
- Felypressin (Octapressin) – since it has similar properties to oxytocin which contracts the uterus, felypressin is contraindicated in pregnant women.

TECHNIQUE OF LOCAL ANAESTHETIC ADMINISTRATION

All dentists should be familiar with local anaesthetic (LA) injection technique both for infiltrating local tissues and for blocking major nerve bundles. Warmed solutions, topical anaesthetic cream and slow injection technique greatly improve patient comfort when injecting LA. Unlike operative dentistry, minor oral surgery also requires palatal, buccal and lingual infiltrations for effective anaesthesia.

COMPLICATIONS OF LOCAL ANAESTHESIA

Local

- Spread of infection through injection into infected tissues.
- Traumatic penetration of nerve (prolonged numbness), vein (haematoma) or artery (systemic toxic effects).
- Tissue damage via pressure necrosis through rapid and forceful injection or withdrawal of bent needle tip through medial pterygoid muscle causing trismus.
- Facial paresis through accidental block of the facial (VII) nerve trunk by a mandibular block being attempted too far posteriorly.

Systemic

- Allergy is rare but is usually related to the methylparaben preservative rather than the LA agent itself.
- Toxicity caused by overdose may lead to unbalanced excitation of the central nervous system (CNS) followed by profound CNS depression with cardiovascular collapse and possibly death.

General anaesthesia

A state of complete unconsciousness.

- **Advantages:**
  excellent for nervous and uncooperative patients
  creates an optimum operating environment for the surgeon who does not have to contend with a restless and constantly moving patient
  complete amnesia for the patient
  permits virtually unlimited operating time
  caters for all degrees of surgical complexity.
- **Disadvantages and limitations:**
  very costly, especially with equipment purchases and maintenance
  the patient must fast for at least 6 hours prior to surgery
  mandatory requirement for expensive monitoring equipment
  requirement for the services of a specialist anaesthetist which significantly adds to the total cost
  postanaesthetic effects demand a recovery bed with close monitoring until the patient regains full consciousness
  general anaesthesia adds significantly to patient inconvenience and the total postoperative morbidity of a surgical procedure
  potentially unsafe for elderly and medically compromised patients.

Technique

There are three phases in the administration of a general anaesthetic agent: induction, maintenance and recovery.

INDUCTION PHASE

The patient is put to sleep using either an inhalation agent or more commonly an intravenously administered anaesthetic induction agent such as methohexitone, thiopentone or propofol.

MAINTENANCE PHASE

The patient is maintained under general anaesthesia with inhalation anaesthetic agents such as halothane, enflurane or isoflurane combined with nitrous oxide.

RECOVERY PHASE

At the completion of surgery, all anaesthetic agents are withdrawn and the patient ventilated with oxygen until consciousness has been regained. The patient is then placed in the recovery position and taken to a recovery area for close monitoring until fully conscious.

Adjunctive measures

For safe general anaesthesia there are important adjunctive measures that need to be considered.

VENTILATION

In the unconscious patient an adequate airway needs to be secured with the provision of an oxygen supply. For simple and quick oral surgical procedures a nasal mask is usually adequate, but for longer operations (>15 minutes) a nasoendotracheal tube is required. Endotracheal intubation is facilitated by the use of various muscle relaxants; however, the use of these agents necessitates assisted positive pressure ventilation until the relaxant is reversed or wears off. Airway protection with an oral or throat pack is mandatory in unconscious patients who have no gag reflex and are in danger of aspirating during oral surgical procedures.

CLOSE MONITORING

It makes sense that there should be two qualified clinicians always present, one to undertake the surgery and the other to closely monitor the anaesthetized patient. Unfortunately, this is not the case in many oral surgery practices in the USA. In this age of high technology, there are various useful gadgets that may assist the anaesthetist in better determining the exact status of the unconscious patient at any given time. Fortunately, the use of the following monitoring equipment is becoming a standard requirement for all general anaesthetic procedures in many countries.

- Pulse oximeter – to monitor oxygen saturation.
- Capnograph – to monitor carbon dioxide excretion.

- Electrocardiograph (ECG) – to monitor regularity and rhythm of heart beat.
- Blood pressure cuff – for intermittent blood pressure measurements.
- Urinary catheter – to monitor fluid balance, particularly for long cases.

LOCAL ANAESTHESIA

The adjunctive use of local anaesthesia during general anaesthesia is commonly undertaken for the following reasons:

to minimize immediate postoperative pain (especially bupivacaine)
to minimize bleeding in the operative field (adrenaline)
to help separate tissue planes for easier dissection
to enable the anaesthetist to maintain the patient on a lighter plane of anaesthesia (i.e. use less anaesthetic drug) since the surgical stimulus is eliminated by the LA.

Sedation

Sedation may be used as an adjunctive measure to local anaesthesia to help improve patient comfort during surgery.

Definition

Sedation is the reduction or abolition of the physiological and psychological responses to the stress of surgery without the loss of consciousness, cooperation or protective reflexes.

Sedation techniques

In minor oral surgery there are three methods of administering sedation:

- Oral – for nervous patients, oral benzodiazepines such as diazepam 2–5 mg may be prescribed the night before and then 1 hour prior to surgery.
- Inhalation – the use of nitrous oxide through a nasal mask is acceptable to many patients; however, adequate sedation is hard to maintain, particularly with natural mouth breathers.
- Intravenous – the most efficient, effective and predictable method of sedation, although it requires experience in venepuncture and some nervous patients are also needle-phobic.

Sedation agents

Benzodiazepines are the most widely used sedation agents; they may be supplemented with short-acting narcotics such as fentanyl for added analgesic effects. The two most commonly used agents are diazepam and midazolam.

DIAZEPAM

Diazepam reduces awareness and anxiety although it has no analgesic properties. It is irritating to peripheral veins and may cause sexual impropriety in some adolescent patients. It is long-acting owing to active metabolites, with a secondary peak 8 hours after the initial dose due to enterohepatic circulation.

Dose: titrate 10–30 mg IV until ptosis or dysarthria.

MIDAZOLAM

Midazolam is twice as potent as diazepam, with a shorter half-life of 2 hours. It is water-soluble, with rapid onset of action after painless injection. Recovery is faster with powerful and predictable anterograde amnesia. Midazolam increases the pain threshold.

Dose: 2.5–7.5 mg IV.

IMPORTANT CONSIDERATIONS

There are three important considerations when sedating a patient:

- Close monitoring – as for general anaesthesia, all sedated patients must be closely monitored with the aid of pulse oximetry and blood pressure measurements during surgery. A portable ECG monitor should ideally be available.
- Airway protection – a sedated patient has a reduced gag reflex so the airway must always be protected with an oral pack placed behind the surgical site.
- Flumazenil is the standard reversal agent for benzodiazepines and must always be available in case of emergency.

Further reading

Brimacombe J, Berry A (1995) The largyngeal mask airway for dental surgery – a review. *Aust Dent J*, **40**, 10–14.

Hill CM, Morris PJ (1991) *General Anaesthesia and Sedation in Dentistry*. 2nd edn. Oxford: Butterworth-Heinemann.

Kippaehne JA, Montgomery MT (1992) Morbidity and mortality from pharmacosedation and general anesthesia in the dental office. *J Oral Maxillofac Surg*, **50**, 691–698.

Loeffler PM (1992) Oral benzodiazepines and conscious sedation: a review. *J Oral Maxillofac Surg*, **50**, 989–997.

Malamed SF (1990) *Handbook of Local Anesthesia*. 3rd edn. St Louis: Mosby YearBook.

4 Simple exodontia

The extraction of teeth is the most important part of minor oral surgery and has the greatest relevance to general dental practice. Although the days of mass dental extractions are long gone, the general dentist will still encounter the need to remove teeth even in fluoridated areas. It is therefore essential that the dental graduate develops and maintains this unique skill of exodontia that no other health professional is trained to do. The aim of this chapter is to introduce the principles and techniques of the simple (intra-alveolar) extraction of teeth.

Terminology

Exodontia – the clinical practice of extracting teeth and tooth fragments.
Intra-alveolar extraction – the removal of teeth from their bony alveolar sockets *without* the need to create a surgical pathway for the delivery of the tooth.
Erupted tooth – where the entire clinical crown of the tooth is visible.

Indications for exodontia

An erupted tooth may be extracted via the intra-alveolar approach for the following reasons.

- **Common reasons:**
    carious tooth that is non-restorable
    periodontally involved tooth that cannot be functionally retained
    non-treatable pulpal or periapical lesion
    to facilitate orthodontic treatment
    significant infection (e.g. cellulitis or abscess)
    patient's informed refusal of restorative treatment (personal prefer-ence or limited time or finances).
- **Uncommon reasons:**
    malpositioned teeth – erupted out of line of arch, difficult to clean and no orthodontic treatment planned
    fractured tooth which is non-restorable, e.g. vertical root fracture
    tooth in line of jaw fracture
    supplementary or supernumerary teeth
    to facilitate the construction of a prosthesis, e.g. lone standing molar

in an otherwise edentulous jaw

teeth associated with pathological lesions, e.g. keratocyst or tumour

prophylactic removal of suspect teeth for patients with major medical conditions, e.g. patients undergoing radiotherapy or heart valve replacement

poor aesthetics – severely stained, eroded, attrited or hypoplastic teeth that cannot be restored.

Contraindications for exodontia

Contraindications are usually relative rather than absolute. Provided the appropriate precautions are taken, teeth may be safely extracted in most situations.

Local factors

Caution is advised in the following situations:

previous radiotherapy to area where tooth is to be removed

teeth in close proximity to tumour (risk of seeding and spread)

acute gingival inflammation with gross plaque and calculus deposits – may result in delayed healing and infection of extraction site.

Systemic factors

Caution is advised in the following situations:

uncontrolled diabetes mellitus

pregnancy

underlying bleeding disorders

acute blood dyscrasias, e.g. leukaemia

cardiac conditions with substantial risk of infective endocarditis

patients on anticoagulants, steroids, immunosuppressants or cancer chemotherapy.

Preoperative evaluation of teeth to be extracted

Prior to extraction, it should be determined whether the tooth in question is suitable for the intra-alveolar approach or whether a surgical approach is warranted from the outset. Factors that favour the intra-alveolar approach are as follows:

- **Clinical factors:**

    good access for instrumentation, e.g. patient with good mouth opening

    periodontally involved teeth

    virtually intact crown

    young patient

    anterior teeth.

- **Radiological factors:**

  simple root configuration, i.e. single, conical root with broad or open apex

  well-defined periodontal space

  loss of alveolar bone height, i.e. advanced periodontal disease

  surrounding alveolar bone of normal texture and free of pathology.

Preparation for simple (intra-alveolar) exodontia

The bare essentials required for simple exodontia are as follows (see Chapters 1–3):

  an informed patient

  basic examination set – dental mirror, dental probe, tweezers and gauze

  strong light and adequate suction

  local anaesthesia, i.e. needle, dental syringe and cartridge of LA solution

  dental extraction instruments:

    dental forceps

    dental elevators.

In addition to the bare essentials the clinician must also have the following on standby:

  dental assistant

  suture set, i.e. needle holder, tissue forceps, cheek retractor and suture

  dental X-ray machine, film and on-site film developing

  a surgical instrument trolley or pack, sterilized and ready to use

  contact telephone number of specialist oral surgeon.

Extraction technique

The most effectively way to extract teeth is to cultivate an efficient technique. A good extraction technique entails two fundamental requirements: adequate access to the tooth, and the use of controlled force to luxate and deliver the tooth.

Adequate access

Access to the tooth is facilitated by the proper positioning of the clinician and the patient (Figure 4.1). For the greatest mechanical advantage, it is best if the clinician is standing up for all extractions. Furthermore, the non-dominant hand (the hand not holding the extraction instrument) should be used to retract the lips and tongue with fingers on either side of the alveolus, and to support the jaw (Figure 4.2).

BRITISH TECHNIQUE

- Forceps are always held with the palm of the hand *above* the handles of the forceps (i.e. the overhand method).

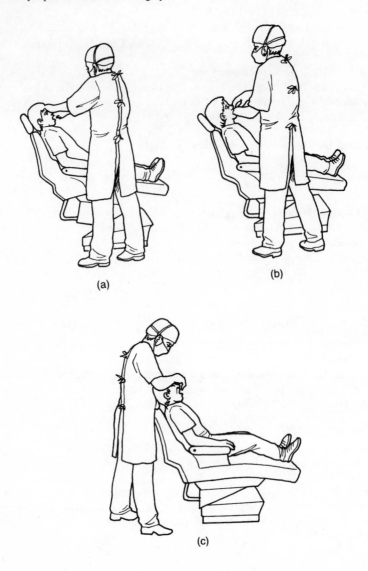

Figure 4.1 Patient–dentist positioning for dental extractions: a, positioning for all extractions in the upper jaw; b, positioning for extractions in the lower left quadrant; c, positioning for extractions in the lower right quadrant.

- The patient is inclined 15–20 degrees for extractions in the lower left quadrant of the mouth and 30–45 degrees for dental extractions in the other three quadrants of the mouth.

- The dentist stands *behind* the patient for extractions in the lower right quadrant of the mouth and in *front* of the patient for all other extractions.

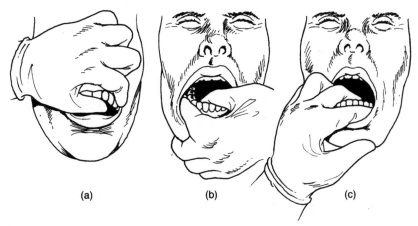

Figure 4.2 Finger positioning and jaw support for dental extractions: a, hand placement for extractions in upper left quadrant; b, hand placement for extractions in the lower right quadrant; c, hand placement for extractions in the lower left quadrant.

NORTH AMERICAN TECHNIQUE

- Forceps are usually held with the palm of the hand *below* the handles of the forceps (i.e. the underhand technique).
- The patient is usually inclined 30–45 degrees for *all* extractions.
- The dentist normally stands *behind* the patient for all extractions.

Use of controlled force

The successful removal of teeth with forceps relies largely on the proper use of controlled force. Excessive force, particularly in awkward directions, can lead to fractures of the crown and hence increase the operating time and surgical morbidity for the patient.

Forceps extractions

The dental forceps are the most commonly used and often the only instruments required for the simple intra-alveolar extraction of teeth.

The basic steps of forceps extractions

1. Grasping the tooth – using the beaks of the forceps to grasp the whole crown of the tooth and part of the root 1–2 mm beyond the cemento-enamel junction.
2. Expansion of the bony socket – see below.
3. Mobilization of the tooth – see below.
4. Delivery of the complete and intact tooth.

The basic forces used to mobilize the tooth

1. Apical pressure – to break the periodontal seal.
2. Buccal force – to expand the buccal plate of bone.
3. Lingual force – to expand the lingual crest of bone.
4. Rotational force – resulting in overall expansion of the tooth socket.
5. Traction force – to deliver the tooth.

Note: always commence with apical pressure and end with traction force to deliver the tooth.

Forceps removal of individual teeth

The extraction technique depends on the tooth being extracted, which is in turn dictated by the morphology of the tooth, in particular its root anatomy. Different teeth not only require different forceps patterns but also emphasis on particular extraction forces which are summarized as follows (Figures 4.3–4.6):

MAXILLARY TEETH

- **Incisors:**
    upper straight forceps
    single conical root pattern
    mainly rotational force required.

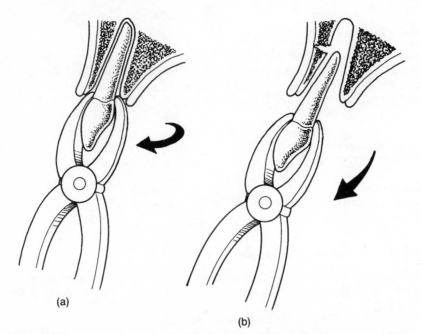

(a)

(b)

Figure 4.3 Forceps extraction of maxillary incisors: a, mainly rotational movement to loosen the tooth within the socket; b, incisor is removed in the buccal direction.

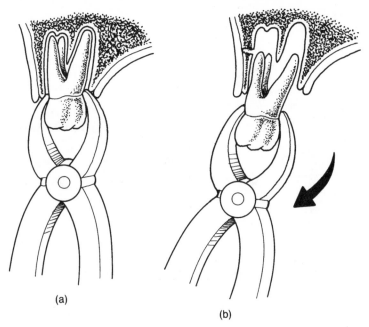

(a)

(b)

Figure 4.4 Forceps extraction of maxillary molars: a, a firm grasp of the crown with anatomical forceps is required; b, extraction is generally achieved in the buccal direction.

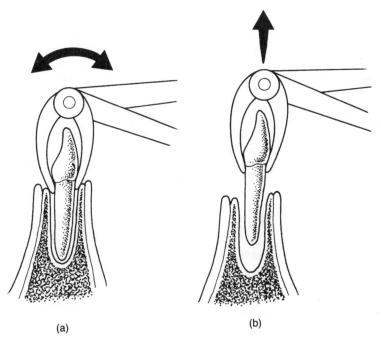

(a)

(b)

Figure 4.5 Forceps extraction of mandibular incisors: a, force is generated in the buccolingual direction; b, the incisor will quickly come once the socket is sufficiently expanded.

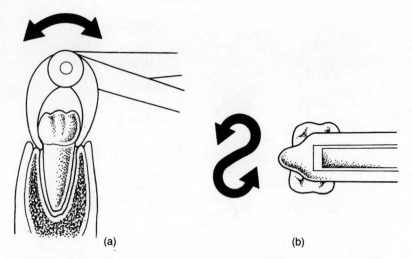

Figure 4.6 Forceps extraction of mandibular molars: a, generally in the buccolingual direction; b, 'figure of eight' movement will help expand the mesial and distal sockets independently.

- **Canines:**
    stubbies
    single long root
    buccopalatal and rotational forces.
- **Premolars:**
    upper universal forceps
    single or double roots which are flattened mesiodistally
    mainly buccolingual movement.
- **Molars:**
    upper left and right hawk's-bill (anatomical) forceps
    three conical roots splayed in triangular configuration
    mainly buccal force.

MANDIBULAR TEETH

- **Incisors:**
    lower universal forceps
    single root flattened mesiodistally
    mainly buccolingual movement.
- **Canines and premolars:**
    lower universal forceps
    single conical roots
    mainly rotational force.
- **Molars:**
    lower hawk's-bill (anatomical) forceps
    two roots flattened mesiodistally
    'figure of eight' movement with buccolingual forces.

The role of dental elevators

Dental elevators sometimes have a role in helping to mobilize teeth prior to the application of the forceps. The Coupland chisels are often used in the initial dilation of the tooth socket and mobilization of the tooth before forceps application. This is particularly useful for teeth adjacent to an edentulous region where the elevator can be successfully used to pry the tooth to be extracted away from its neighbouring tooth, providing greater access for the beaks of the forceps to be applied. Dental elevators play a much larger role in the surgical extraction of teeth and tooth fragments (see Chapters 5–7).

Further reading

Howe GL (1990) *The Extraction of Teeth.* 2nd edn. Oxford: Butterworth-Heinemann.

Moore JR, Gillbe GV (1991) *Principles of Oral Surgery.* 4th edn, pp 75–92. Manchester University Press.

Peterson LJ, Ellis III E, Hupp JR, Tucker MR (1993) *Contemporary Oral and Maxillofacial Surgery.* 2nd edn, pp 132–185. St Louis: Mosby.

5 Surgical exodontia

All dental practitioners should be conversant with the principles of surgical exodontia, which is employed for the management of difficult erupted teeth, retained roots and impacted teeth. Surgical exodontia should not be undertaken lightly, and unless the clinician has had the opportunity to develop his or her surgical skills under supervised instruction, then general dental practice is not the place to start. The aim of this chapter is to introduce the basic principles of surgical exodontia.

Terminology

Surgical exodontia – the removal of teeth or tooth fragments via the transalveolar approach, whereby access to and delivery of the tooth or its fragments are achieved via a surgically created pathway.
Transalveolar approach – where the alveolar bone and soft tissues surrounding the tooth or its fragments are surgically breached to create a pathway required to undertake a surgical exodontia.
Difficult erupted teeth – teeth with crowns fully visible in the mouth, which – for whatever reason – cannot be completely removed by the intra-alveolar approach alone.
Impacted tooth – a tooth that fails to erupt, for whatever reason, into the dental arch within the expected time frame.

The basic steps of surgical exodontia

The surgical extraction of teeth and tooth fragments consists of six fundamental steps:

1. Raising a flap.
2. Removal of bone.
3. Tooth division.
4. Removal of tooth or tooth fragments.
5. Wound toilet.
6. Primary closure.

Not all surgical extractions need to go through each of the six steps. In many cases, a tooth may be surgically extracted simply by raising a flap without having to remove bone or divide the tooth.

Raising a flap

A flap is a tongue of tissue comprising a base and a distal segment which is raised from its surrounding tissue bed.

FUNCTION

A flap serves two fundamental purposes:

to provide access to the surgical site
to serve as the primary dressing to cover the surgical defect that is created.

TYPES

Many types of flaps are used in surgery, but in minor oral surgery the most common is a mucoperiosteal flap, i.e. oral mucosa and periosteum that cover the alveolar process.

Flaps may be described in terms of their physical shape or outline, or more often according to the site from which the flap is procured, e.g. buccal flap, palatal flap or lingual flap.

TECHNICAL NOTES

1. The incision must be made in one continuous stroke through to bone at right angles to the surface of the mucosa.
2. The base of the flap, where the blood supply is derived, must always be wider than its distal segment in order to maintain the viability of the flap when it is raised from its tissue bed (Figure 5.1).

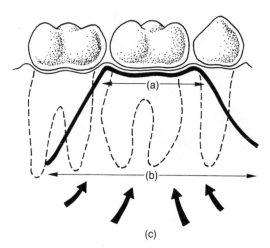

Figure 5.1 Flap outline. The margin of the base of the flap (b) must be wider than the distal segment (a) since the blood supply (c) is derived from the base of the flap.

3. The dental papilla should always be wholly included on the distal margin of the flap and not split, to avoid poor gingival contours after healing.
4. Once raised with the aid of a periosteal elevator, the flap must be handled gently to avoid stretching and tearing of its margins which will compromise its healing potential.
5. The edges of the flap must alway lie on sound bone at the end of the operative procedure in order to prevent wound dehiscence and break-down.

Removal of bone

Bone is removed (Figure 5.2) to expose enough tooth in order to:

permit the application of dental elevators
allow adequate exposure for sectioning of the tooth
provide an adequate pathway for delivery of the tooth or tooth fragments.

INSTRUMENTATION

Bone may be removed by the use of sharp chisels, or powered handpieces with round or fissured surgical burrs; these are water-cooled with the exhaust facing away from the surgical site. High-speed air turbines may

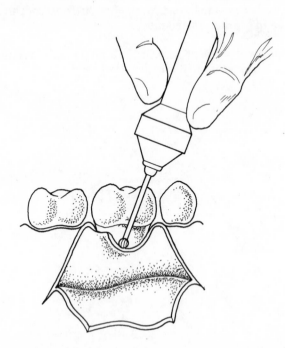

Figure 5.2 Bone removal via guttering technique. This will help expose enough root surface to allow the purchase of elevators or division of the tooth. Best achieved with a round surgical burr.

create surgical wound emphysema (see Chapter 14) and do not allow enough tactile discrimination between bone and tooth substance.

Tooth division

It is particularly useful to section teeth in the following cases:

where the awkward angulation or position of the tooth does not permit its delivery in one piece
where smaller fragments can be easily lifted out of the bony socket, thereby minimizing the need to remove further bone.

INSTRUMENTATION

Teeth can be sectioned using either an osteotome, which is quick but the split is often unpredictable, or a powered handpiece, which is slow but more predictable (Figure 5.3).

TECHNICAL NOTE

The direction in which the tooth is divided – axial, coronal, vertical or horizontal – depends on:

the angulation of the tooth
the number and pattern of the roots
the path of delivery of the tooth or its individual fragments.

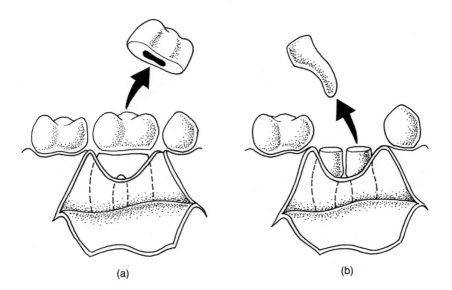

(a)   (b)

Figure 5.3 Tooth division: a, using a jet or tapered fissure burr, the crown is first separated and removed from the roots; b, the roots are then divided and removed individually.

Removal of tooth or tooth fragments

The removal of the tooth or tooth fragments constitutes the most important part of the whole surgical exercise (Figure 5.4). Successful removal is
largely dependent on:

- The quality of the surgical access created – i.e. has enough bone been
  removed to expose the site for the application of a dental elevator?
- The correct use of the dental elevators – a suitable point of purchase or
  fulcrum is needed for the instrument to be used in a rotating motion to
  luxate the tooth or tooth roots.

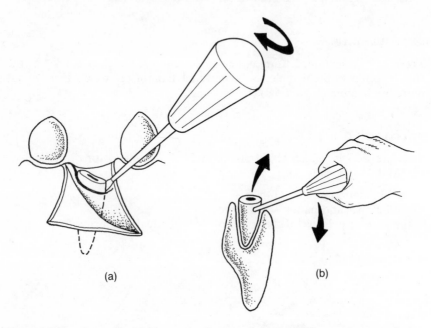

(a)   (b)

Figure 5.4 Elevating a root fragment: a, application of a straight elevator to remove a root.
Note the angle of the instrument and the twisting motion used to subluxate the root from
the socket; b, by placing the tip of the elevator into a prepared hole within the coronal part
of the root, the root may be subluxated using the crestal margin of alveolar bone as a
fulcrum.

Wound toilet

After the whole tooth or all the tooth fragments have been completely
removed, the remaining surgical defect must be thoroughly debrided and
irrigated to remove all loose debris that may cause infections and delay
wound healing. Wound toilet may involve:

1. Excising redundant soft tissue, e.g. remnant of dental follicle.
2. Removing any loose fragments of bone or tooth in and around the surgical defect, including under the flap.
3. Smoothing rough bony edges with burr or bone files.

4. Irrigating with sterile isotonic solution (saline) and suctioning the area to remove microscopic debris.
5. On occasions, the surgical defect may be sprinkled with antibiotic powder or dressed with antiseptic-soaked ribbon gauze.

Primary closure

The surgical defect must be sealed from the oral environment by replacement of the flap and careful suturing to permit well-approximated wound margins without tension. The flap acts as the primary dressing and contains the osteogenic layer of periosteum which will help promote bone regeneration within the surgical defect. The type of suture used is a matter of surgeon preference. For patient convenience, however, resorbable sutures are preferable (see Chapter 1).

Surgical extraction of erupted teeth

Indications

A surgical approach for the extraction of erupted teeth should always be considered when the following situations are encountered:

patient with a history of difficult extractions
patient is a large, adult male of African or southern Mediterranean descent
a tooth that resists forceps extraction
grossly carious tooth with significant likelihood of fracturing upon application of dental forceps
a tooth that has been subjected to trauma – fracture of roots or alveolar bone
lone standing maxillary molar – especially in middle-aged or elderly patients
radiographic evidence of complex root patterns, bulbous root apex, ankylosis, hypercementosis or dense alveolar bone texture
endodontically treated teeth – often very brittle.

Technical notes

1. Always obtain an updated preoperative radiograph of the tooth in question before commencing surgery.
2. When outlining a flap, try to avoid incising the gingival margins of adjacent teeth; confine the gingival margin incision to the tooth being extracted with a mesial and/or distal relieving incision for greater access.
3. Make sure the flap margins lie on sound bone and not over the surgical defect.
4. Dividing the tooth will help minimize the removal of alveolar bone necessary to allow delivery of the tooth.
5. Alveolar bone removal should be conservative, with the aim of providing a solid purchase point for the most effective application of the dental elevators.

Retained or fractured root

The presence of a retained or fractured root is not in itself an indication for removal, particularly where the likely morbidity of the surgery outweighs the benefits gained from the removal of the root, e.g. paraesthesia following the removal of an asymptomatic root fragment close to the inferior dental canal.

FACTORS PREDISPOSING TO ROOT FRACTURES DURING DENTAL EXTRACTIONS

- History of difficult extractions.
- Extensively restored teeth, especially those that are non-vital and root-filled.
- Deep cervical caries.
- Complex root pattern with multiple and in particular, fine roots.
- Dense bone, hypercementosis and ankylosis.
- Clumsy use of excessive force to extract tooth.

It is important ALWAYS to inspect the root tips of all extracted teeth to ensure that fracture of the thin apices has not occurred.

INDICATIONS FOR THE REMOVAL OF RETAINED ROOTS

- Pulpal pathology – non-vital roots.
- Periapical pathology – infection, granuloma, cyst.
- Likelihood of exposure with progressive alveolar bone resorption.
- Planned orthodontics or fixed prosthesis.

If fractured roots are to be left in situ, they should be recorded and the patient informed.

TECHNICAL NOTES

1. Multiple X-ray views with the aid of radio-opaque markers may be required to locate small fragments.
2. Examination of the extracted teeth will indicate the size and shape of the fractured root.
3. Before embarking on surgical removal, the potential morbidity must be considered in terms of the proximity of the root fragment to:
   the maxillary sinus floor
   the inferior dental canal
   potential tissue spaces such as the pterygopalatine fossa.
4. In an edentulous alveolus, the safest incision is along the crest of the ridge with a mesial releiving incision if greater access is required.
5. Bone removal should be planned to minimize the effect on the healed ridge form, i.e. every attempt should be made to preserve the height and width of the alveolar ridge.

Impacted teeth

Aetiology

The path of eruption is impeded by:

crowded adjacent teeth or not enough room in the dental arch
dense overlying bone
excessive soft tissue
retained and ankylosed deciduous teeth
pathology – supernumerary teeth, odontomas, cysts.

In some cases impactions may be the result of stunted growth secondary to irradiation or a developmental anomaly such as cleidocranial dysplasia.

Occurrence

The most commonly impacted teeth, in descending order of frequency, are:

mandibular third molars
maxillary third molars
maxillary canines
mandibular premolars.

The surgical management of impacted teeth is discussed in more detail in Chapters 6 and 7.

Further reading

Amier HA (1977) The age factor in human extraction wound healing. *J Oral Surg*, **35**, 193–197.
Howe GL (1985) *Minor Oral Surgery*. 3rd edn, pp 92–108. Oxford: Butterworth-Heinemann.
Koerner KR, Tilt LV, Johnson KR (1994) *Color Atlas of Minor Oral Surgery*. London: Mosby-Wolfe.
Moore JR, Gillbe GV (1991) *Principles of Oral Surgery*. 4th edn, pp 75–92. Manchester University Press.
Peterson LJ, Ellis III E, Hupp JR, Tucker MR (1993) *Contemporary Oral and Maxillofacial Surgery*. 2nd edn, pp 186–224. St Louis: Mosby.

6 Mandibular third molars

The evolutionary decrease in jaw size is reflected by the modern human diet of relatively soft processed foods. With the reduced jaw dimensions there is insufficient space within the dental arch for the mandibular third molars which are consequently the most frequently impacted of all teeth in the human jaws. Eruption times for mandibular third molars vary enormously and are often unpredictable, particularly in cases where the individual is fortunate to have maintained the full complement of their permanent dentition into early adulthood. The surgical removal of mandibular third molars constitutes a substantial part of the dental health expenditure of most affluent nations, and will continue to do so well into the twenty-first century. All dental practitioners should therefore develop a protocol for the surgical removal of third molars, bearing in mind the controversies surrounding the prophylactic removal of asymptomatic wisdom teeth that surface in the literature and the media from time to time.

Indications for removal

The indications for the surgical removal of mandibular third molars are as follows:

- **Common reasons** (in descending order of frequency):
  pericoronitis (see Chapter 8)
  prophylactic removal of symptomless teeth, frequently for orthodontic reasons (see note below)
  caries
  periodontal disease – deep pocketing along distal root of lower second molar.
- **Uncommon reasons:**
  previous failed attempted extraction elsewhere
  associated pathology, e.g. cysts or more rarely tumours
  exposure under denture
  obscure facial pain.

Note: there is much controversy concerning the prophylactic removal of asymptomatic impacted third molars. Guidelines have been established by specialist groups in a number of countries. Since these guidelines vary from country to country and may change from time to time, readers are advised to consult the most recent guidelines published within their own country of practice.

Radiological investigations

An adequate and up-to-date radiograph (preferably less than 6 months old) is the single most important clinical aid in surgical planning. The orthopantomogram is an excellent screening film that is safe and reliable and has now become the standard radiograph for the preoperative radiological assessment for all third molar surgery.

While it is essential to have adequate radiographs of the symptomatic teeth clinically visible in the oral cavity, it is equally important to investigate the presence of other impacted teeth or jaw pathology that may be dealt with at the same operation. In many instances where the removal of third molars is planned, particularly under general anaesthesia, it may be considered negligent on the clinician's part not to obtain an adequate orthopantomogram prior to surgery.

Assessing surgical difficulty

Once the decision has been made to remove the mandibular third molar or molars, the next step is to ascertain the degree of difficulty that may be encountered in the surgical removal of the tooth in question. The degree of surgical difficulty has important implications not only in the surgical approach but also in the management of the patient, for instance whether it is necessary to supplement local anaesthesia with sedation for greater patient comfort and compliance. The degree of surgical difficulty in the removal of mandibular third molars is dependent upon the following factors.

Access

Access is the most important indicator of difficulty. Patients with restricted mouth opening for whatever reason are by far the most difficult cases for the removal of mandibular third molars.

Root pattern

The optimal time for removal of mandibular third molars is when the root is only two-thirds developed.

In the early teenage years, when no roots are present and only the crown is formed, surgical removal of the mandibular third molar is complicated by the absence of a stable purchase point, as the crown rolls freely around in its crypt.

In mature adults where the root apices are fully developed, the degree of surgical difficulty increases with the number of roots and increasing complexity of the root pattern and morphology.

Degree of eruption

An erupted tooth offers a purchase point for dental elevators without the need to raise flaps, therefore simplifying the surgery.

An unerupted tooth requires raising a flap for access and may even necessitate bone removal depending on the degree of impaction, hence increasing the complexity of the surgery.

Depth of impaction

The deeper the impaction, the more bone must be removed in order to gain access to the tooth, increasing the morbidity, complexity and duration of the operation.

Angulation of tooth

The least difficult teeth are often those where the long axis of the tooth is vertical (or perpendicular) with respect to the mandibular occlusal plane. In some cases, however, vertical functioning teeth with complex root patterns may prove difficult to remove.

Where the tooth is tilted mesially or distally, or lies horizontal (or parallel) with respect to the mandibular occlusal plane, the degree of surgical difficulty increases. This is because the path of removal is obstructed by either the second molar or alveolar bone.

Age of the patient

Generally speaking, the older the patient, the more difficult the surgery. This is mainly due to the increase in density and decreased elasticity of the bone with age which necessitates greater bone removal and increased potential morbidity of the surgery.

Sex and race

Large men, particularly of southern European or Afro-Caribbean stock, tend to be difficult cases.

Small women also tend to present problems of restricted access due to small mouths and limited mouth opening.

Classification of mandibular third molar impactions

Classification of third molar impactions is necessary for the sake of clear communication between clinicians and adequate record-keeping which may be used for audit or research purposes. Mandibular third molar impactions may be classified according to the degree of impaction, angulation of the tooth and proximity to the inferior alveolar canal (Figure 6.1).

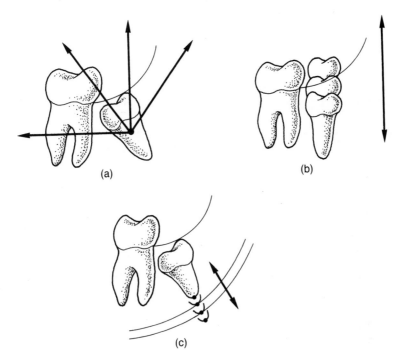

Figure 6.1 Classification of lower third molar impactions: a, angulation of the tooth – direction of impaction according to the inclination or angulation of the long axis of the tooth relative to the occlusal plane; b, degree of impaction – depth of impaction relative to the external oblique ridge; c, proximity to the inferior alveolar canal – relationship of the inferior alveolar canal to the apex of the mandibular third molar.

Degree of impaction

1. No impaction – *fully erupted tooth which may be in*
   (a) functional occlusion with tooth in opposing arch *or*
   (b) non-functional.
2. Soft tissue impaction
   (a) partly erupted tooth
   (b) unerupted tooth.
3. Bony impaction – *unerupted tooth with crown that may be*
   (a) partially surrounded by bone
   (b) totally surrounded by bone.

Angulation of the tooth

Tooth angulation in the sagittal and transverse planes may be classified as:

1. Vertical
   (a) buccoversion
   (b) linguoversion.

2. Mesioangular
   (a) buccoversion
   (b) linguoversion.
3. Distoangular
   (a) buccoversion
   (b) linguoversion.
4. Horizontal
   (a) buccoversion
   (b) linguoversion.
5. Heterotopic – the tooth is found in unusual places along the lower border of the mandible or high up the ascending ramus, usually in an inverted position.

Proximity to the inferior alveolar canal

1. No contact.
2. Root apices in direct contact.
3. Roots crossing canal on one side only – no imprint of canal on root surface.
4. Roots partially encircling canal – imprint of canal clearly visible on root surface.
5. Roots completely encircling canal – canal passes between the roots of the tooth.

Note: radiographs can only project a two-dimensional image of the three-dimensional relationship between the roots of the mandibular third molar and the inferior alveolar canal. Radiographics clues that may indicate physical contact between the roots and the canal include:

   decrease in the width of the canal as it crosses the roots
   decrease in the radio-opacity of the roots as they cross the canal
   sudden change in direction of the canal as it crosses the roots
   loss of one or both radio-opaque boundaries of the canal as it crosses the roots.

Operative technique

The surgical removal of mandibular third molars follows the basic principles of surgical exodontia as described in Chapter 5.

Raising a flap

There are four incisions that can be used to raise a flap when extracting mandibular third molars (Figure 6.2).

DISTAL RELIEVING INCISION

A distobuccal incision is made along the anterior border of the ascending ramus. The simplest flaps can be raised with this incision alone. Most

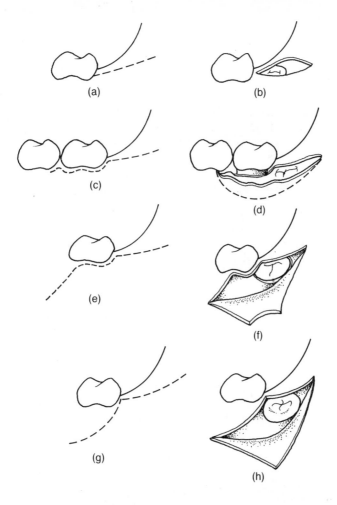

Figure 6.2 Flap design for lower third molars: a, distal relieving incision; b, limited exposure offered by distal relieving incision; c, envelope flap; d, still quite limited exposure with envelope flap; e, buccal extension flap; f, greater exposure offered with buccal extension flap; g, triangular flap; h, excellent exposure without the need to involve the gingival margins of the adjacent teeth when using a triangular flap.

often used where the distal part of the crown is covered by soft tissue such as the operculum.

ENVELOPE FLAP

The anterior incision is extended forwards along the gingival crevice of the second and first molar as far as the mesial interproximal papilla of the first molar.

- **Disadvantages:**
    provides limited access for deep impactions

if postoperative infection occurs, the gingival crevice may break down creating periodontal pockets along the first and second molars.

BUCCAL EXTENSION FLAP

The incision along the gingival crevice is confined to the second molar with a buccal relieving incision extending inferiorly and anteriorly from the mesial or halfway along the second molar down to the vestibular sulcus in a gentle arc. Access is much greater although potential periodontal problems are still present.

TRIANGULAR FLAP

A triangular flap that keeps well away from the gingival attachment of adjacent teeth and sweeps down and forwards from the distal surface of the second molar into the mucobuccal fold gives good access without the potential periodontal problems.

Removal of bone

Bone surrounding the tooth may be removed in one of a number of ways (Figure 6.3).

LINGUAL SPLIT TECHNIQUE

Despite the advantages of speed, rapid healing and the requirement for only simple instrumentation, the lingual split technique is now merely of historical interest in most countries outside Great Britain. The major

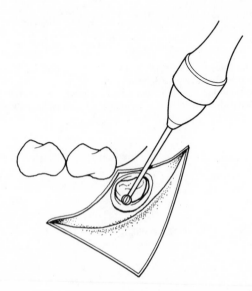

Figure 6.3 Bone removal. A round burr is used to remove bone largely on the buccal aspect.

disadvantages are the requirement for large flaps, removal of large segments of lingual bone plate and the increased potential risk of injury to the lingual nerve.

BUCCAL APPROACH

Using a high-powered handpiece with a round surgical burr, bone removal is confined to the buccal aspect where a bone gutter is created around the tooth to expose the maximum convexity of the crown so as to create a point of application for the dental elevators. This is a conservative approach, the purpose of which is to minimize the amount of bone removal with greater emphasis on tooth division; the latter is achieved using tapered fissure burrs (see below).

EXTENDED BUCCAL APPROACH

In many instances, distal bone may be drilled away using a periosteal elevator to carefully retract and protect the lingual tissues from the point of the burr. Although this approach provides greater tooth exposure and lessens the need for tooth division, there is an increased risk of lingual nerve damage due to stretching of the retracted lingual tissues.

Sectioning teeth

The most difficult part of mandibular third molar surgery is understanding the most mechanically advantageous way of dividing a tooth according to its impaction (Figure 6.4).

VERTICAL IMPACTIONS

The tooth is best divided in half along its vertical axis and each half removed individually.

HORIZONTAL IMPACTIONS

The crown is separated from its roots and removed first. The roots are themselves divided and removed individually into the space vacated by the crown.

MESIOANGULAR IMPACTIONS

The tooth may be divided in half along its longitudinal axis or the crown may be divided obliquely with the distal segment removed first prior to mobilizing the rest of the tooth.

DISTOANGULAR IMPACTIONS

The tooth may be divided in half along its longitudinal axis or the crown may be sectioned from its roots with the roots being elevated into the space vacated by the crown.

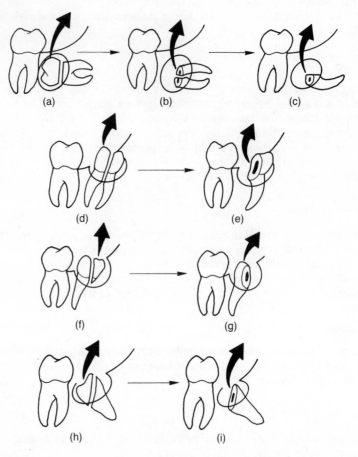

Figure 6.4 Dividing lower third molars: a, horizontal impaction – crown is sectioned and removed first; b, roots are sectioned – upper root removed first; c, lower root is removed last; d, distoangular impactions – tooth is divided along its long axis; e, removal of the mesial portion creates room for the distal fragment to be moved into for extraction, thereby avoiding sacrifice of further distal bone; f, for single-rooted teeth, splitting the bulky crown will facilitate removal; g, removal of tooth is easy when the crown is substantially reduced in size; h, oblique sectioning of crown and its removal; i, with the crown gone, the root can be subluxated into the space vacated by the crown.

Wound toilet

It is important to irrigate the surgical site, with particular attention paid to the space directly underneath the buccal flap where loose debris may accumulate and cause a buccal space infection. Adequate haemostasis is also important prior to wound closure to minimize the risk of persistent post-operative oozing and haematoma formation.

Closure

The most important suture is the one placed immediately behind the second molar, ensuring there is accurate apposition of wound edges (Figure 6.5). It is also useful to place a suture across the distal incision where the soft tissue thickness and potential bleeding source is greatest. Many clinicians often do not place sutures across the buccal relieving incision, which permits a dependent area of drainage. Water-tight closure is unnecessary and may in some cases increase postoperative pain and swelling. Resorbable sutures are often more convenient for the patient as access to remove non-resorbable sutures is limited in this area of the mouth and the exercise may be distressing to the patient only a week after surgery.

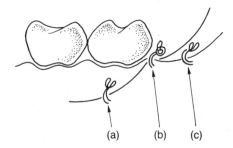

(a)   (b)   (c)

Figure 6.5 Wound closure: a, the mesial suture is optional and often not required; b, the distolingual suture is the most important suture of all and must be carefully and securely placed immediately behind the second molar; c, the distobuccal suture, although optional, is often important particularly for haemorrhage control.

Further reading

Alling III CC, Helfrick JF, Alling RD (1993) *Impacted Teeth*. Philadelphia: Saunders.
Eliasson S, Heimdahl A, Nordenram A (1989) Pathological changes related to long term impaction of third molars. A radiographic study. *Int J Oral Maxillofac Surg*, **18**, 210–212.
Koerner KR, Tilt LV, Johnson KR (1994) *Color Atlas of Minor Oral Surgery*. London: Mosby-Wolfe.
Lopes V, Mumenya R, Feinmann C, Harris M (1995) Third molar surgery: an audit of the indications for surgery, post-operative complaints and patient satisfaction. *Br J Oral Maxillofac Surg*, **33**, 33–35.
Lysell L, Rohlin M (1988) A study of indications used for removal of the mandibular third molar. *Int J Oral Maxillofac Surg*, **17**, 161–164.
Mercier P, Precious D (1992) Risks and benefits of removal of impacted third molars: a critical review of the literature. *J Oral Maxillofac Surg*, **21**, 17–27.
Rood JP (1983) Lingual split technique; damage to inferior alveolar and lingual nerves during removal of impacted mandibular third molars. *Br Dent J*, **154**, 402.
Tetsch P, Wagner W (1985) *Operative Extraction of Wisdom Teeth*. London: Wolfe.

7 Other impacted teeth

Less commonly impacted teeth include the maxillary third molars, the maxillary canines and the mandibular premolars (in descending order of frequency). In this chapter the clinical presentation and surgical management of these impacted teeth is discussed.

Terminology

Transplantation – the transferring of a living organ or tissue from one part of the body to another, within the same individual (autogenic), between different individuals of the same species (allogenic), or between different species (xenogenic).

Maxillary third molars

When present, the maxillary third molars are often extracted at the same time as the mandibular third molars since they are seldom of any functional value even when they are fully erupted.

Indications for removal

- **Erupted teeth:**
    non-functional – due to impaction of opposing lower third molar
    supererupted or buccally displaced – causing direct trauma to operculum surrounding partially erupted lower third molar
    difficult to clean – due to restricted access for toothbrushing
    caries
    periodontal disease.
- **Unerupted teeth** (often asymptomatic):
    lack of space in the dental arch for eruption into a functional position
    patient convenience – to have maxillary third molars removed at the same time as removal of mandibular third molars
    resorption of adjacent maxillary second molars
    associated pericoronal pathology – dentigerous cyst, odontogenic tumour, etc.

Investigations

Radiographs are essential in planning the surgical management of maxillary third molars. The two most commonly used radiographs are described below.

PERIAPICAL X-RAYS

Periapical X-rays are simple and cost-effective. Location of an impacted upper third molar, however, makes positioning of the film and the central beam of the X-ray very much a hit and miss affair, which may necessitate multiple exposures to capture the whole tooth on film.

ORTHOPANTOMOGRAM

The orthopantomogram is an excellent screening film that includes all third molars on the one film. Furthermore, there is a broader appreciation of each impacted tooth in relation to its surrounding anatomy. It is the view of choice, particularly where multiple impacted teeth are present.

Surgical planning

The difficulty of maxillary third molar surgery lies not in the angulation of the impaction or the complexity of the roots, but rather in how high up the posterior maxilla the tooth is found. When maxillary third molars are considered in isolation, the degree of surgical difficulty may be considered from three levels (Figure 7.1).

- First level – the tooth is erupted or partially erupted. These teeth are easily removed under local anaesthesia alone with relatively little morbidity.
- Second level – the tooth is unerupted but the crown margin of the tooth is below the level of the apices of the second molar tooth. Although a surgical approach is required, the tooth is still easily accessible to dental elevators and may require no more than local anaesthesia and IV sedation.

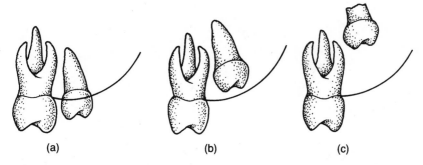

(a)   (b)   (c)

Figure 7.1 Classification of upper third molar impactions: a, first level; b, second level; c, third level.

- Third level – when the crown of the unerupted maxillary third molar is above the apices of the adjacent second molar tooth, the degree of impaction poses the greatest surgical difficulty of all. In some cases, general anaesthesia may be required to gain wider and greater access to the tooth which harbours an increased likelihood of being accidentally displaced into the maxillary antrum or infratemporal fossa.

Note: it is often the case that the decision between local anaesthesia and general anaesthesia is based on the degree of difficulty of the mandibular third molars rather than the maxillary third molars.

Surgical technique

The technique used to extract maxillary third molars depends on the position of the tooth.

ERUPTED TEETH

The procedure begins with buccal and palatal infiltration of local anaesthetic solution.

A straight or curved elevator is placed within the interproximal area between the second and third molar.

Twisting the elevator in the buccodistal direction will luxate the tooth sufficiently for the tooth to be removed with the fingers which should be straddling the socket (Figure 7.2).

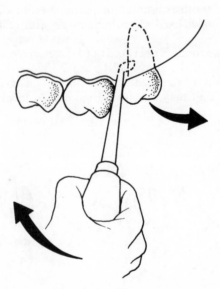

Figure 7.2 Extraction of upper third molars with dental elevators. Note the curved elevator placed interproximally which is twisted to luxate the upper third molar in the distobuccal direction.

Upper curved (bayonet) forceps may also be used to extract erupted maxillary third molars with the force concentrated mainly in the buccal direction.

Make sure the airway is protected or else the luxated tooth may accidentally be lost in the pharynx, with the danger of it being aspirated (see Chapter 14).

PARTLY ERUPTED TEETH

The procedure is the same as for a fully erupted tooth, except that a small mesial and/or distal relieving incision may be required for better instrument access and to prevent tearing of the gingiva as the tooth is luxated.

UNERUPTED TEETH

The flap outline consists of a distal and mesial incision which may vary as follows:

- **Distal incision** – made behind the distal surface of the second molar:
    sagitally along the maxillary tuberosity
    diagonally across the maxillary tuberosity.
- **Mesial incision** – made across the buccal attached gingiva of the adjacent second molar:
    along the gingival crevice – which has restricted access to low impactions
    diagonally upward relieving incision – which may be extended according to the height of the impaction to provide good access (Figure 7.3).

A full mucoperiosteal flap is raised using a periosteal elevator.

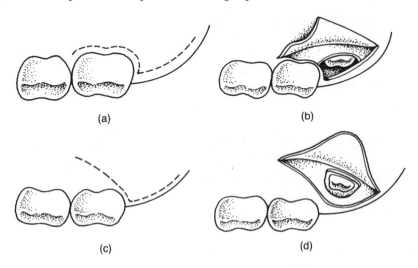

(a)

(b)

(c)

(d)

Figure 7.3 Flap design for upper third molars: a, b, mesial incision made along gingival margin gives good access for low impactions; c, d, superiorly extended mesial incision gives good access for high impactions.

An instrument such as a periosteal elevator or a Laster's retractor should be placed behind the bony tuberosity to prevent backward displacement of the tooth during luxation.

Bone removal is facilitated by the soft membranous nature of posterior maxillary bone, so that chisels can be used to chip away the thin buccal plate of bone covering the unerupted tooth.

Once the tooth is adequately exposed, a fine curved elevator, such as a curved Warwick-James, is placed across the mesial surface of the third molar in the interproximal space between it and the distal surface of the second molar.

Rotation of the elevator will effectively luxate the tooth in the bucco-distal direction, so a protective posteriorly placed retractor will help the delivery of the tooth in a buccal direction.

Thorough wound toilet is essential, ensuring there is no oroantral communication (see Chapter 10), followed by primary closure with sutures across the distal and mesial incisions. Some clinicians do not place any sutures since the cheek itself holds the flap in place.

Maxillary canines

Maxillary canines should be palpable in the alveolus by 8–9 years of age. If the canine has not erupted by 12 years of age then it is the dentist's responsibility to check and see where it is.

Causes of maxillary canine impaction

1. Non-resorption of deciduous canine.
2. Ankylosis of impacted canine.
3. Contracted or collapsed maxillary arch.
4. Absence of lateral incisor to guide canines into the arch.
5. Presence of pathology, supernumerary teeth or scar tissue in the path of eruption.
6. Trauma – disturbance of the tooth germ axis.

Sequelae

If the impacted canine is left in situ it may result in one or more of the following sequelae (Figure 7.4):

resorption of adjacent lateral incisor roots
dentigerous cyst formation
infection – if there is communication with the oral cavity.

Clinical presentation

1. Obvious firm bulge in buccal alveolus or palate.
2. Distal inclination of lateral incisor – due to impacted canine hitting against its roots.

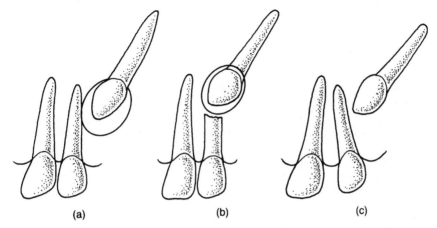

Figure 7.4 Radiographic presentation of impacted maxillary canines: a, cyst formation; b, resorption of adjacent lateral incisor root; c, distal tipping of lateral incisor.

Radiographic examination

Radiographic determination of the position of the tooth is required in order to plan the surgical approach – buccal (20%) or palatal (80%). The dentist has a choice of one or more of the following radiographic techniques:

- Vertex occlusal view – to show either buccal or palatal displacement.
- Parallax method – using the tube shift technique with two periapical films. If the canine moves in the same direction as the tube shift, then it is palatally placed.
- Orthopantomograph – demonstrates the vertical and mesiodistal relationship of the canine and also the inclination of its long axis relative to the other teeth.
- Lateral skull view – will show the vertical height and the anteroposterior position of the canine relative to the other teeth.
- Posteroanterior skull view – provides additional information about the position of the canine in the transverse dimension.

Factors that influence treatment planning

1. The degree of crowding or spacing in the arch.
2. Degree of displacement of the canine.
3. Attitude of the patient or the patient's parents.
4. Oral hygiene standard, age and compliance of patient.
5. Root morphology of canine.
6. Any associated pathology:
     in the canine itself
     in the eruption path of the canine
     in the adjacent teeth.

Treatment options

- **Leave in situ:**

    asymptomatic canine where surgery is likely to cause damage to adjacent teeth

    informed refusal of patient for surgical treatment

    elderly, frail, medically compromised or terminally ill patients.

- **Surgical exposure:**

    if performed after the active eruptive phase of the maxillary canine (i.e. patient over 12 years old) then orthodontically assisted traction is required to bring the tooth into position

    eruption path free of obstructions

    adequate space in the arch is naturally present or will be created orthodontically

    favourable (i.e. vertical) inclination of the long axis of the canine.

- **Extract canine:**

    adjacent teeth are being damaged by the presence of the impacted canine, e.g. root resorption

    other surgical options impractical because of:

    apical curvature of root

    deep or awkward position of impacted canine

    time factor

    poor patient compliance

    severe lack of space in the arch

    good prognosis for retained deciduous canine

    pathology associated with impacted canine, e.g. dentigerous cyst.

- **Transplant canine:**

    best reserved as a last resort

    prognosis is dependent on careful surgical technique

    adequate space in the arch to accommodate the transplanted tooth is essential.

Surgical extraction of the impacted maxillary canine

Make sure there is enough clinical and radiographic data available to determine the easiest and most accessible approach to the impacted tooth before commencing surgery.

BUCCAL APPROACH

The buccal approach is used in 20% of cases (Figure 7.5).

1. Raise a mucoperiosteal flap over the buccal alveolus.
2. Remove bone to expose the crown beyond its greatest convexity.
3. Because it is such a large tooth, the canine is often divided and the crown is removed separately from the root.
4. Wound toilet.
5. Flap closed with interdental sutures.

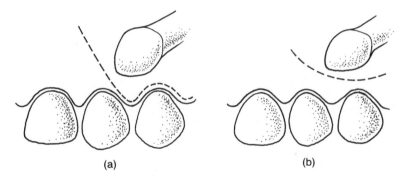

Figure 7.5 Buccal flap approach to impacted maxillary canines: a, gingival margin incision; b, semilunar incision.

PALATAL APPROACH

The palatal approach (Figure 7.6) is used in 80% of cases.

1. Gingival margin incision is made extending from the second premolar on one side to the second premolar on the opposite side of the palate.
2. Carefully raise a full-thickness palatal flap.
3. Sharply dissect the incisive neurovascular bundle at the incisive foramen.
4. Remove bone to uncover the crown beyond its greatest convexity and expose at least the coronal part of the root.

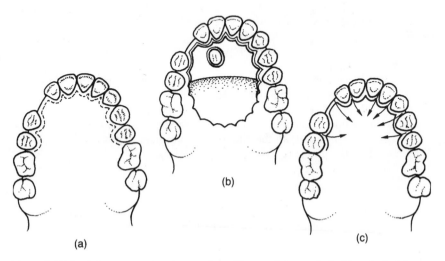

Figure 7.6 Palatal flap approach to impacted maxillary canines: a, gingival margin incision extending from second premolar to second premolar; b, palatal mucoperiosteal flap raised and bone removed to expose crown of impacted canine; c, closure with interdental sutures taking deep bites of the palatal flap to prevent haematoma formation under the flap.

5. It is often necessary to divide and separately remove the crown from the root. The removal of the crown first allows room for the root to be luxated into prior to either removal or further division.
6. Wound toilet.
7. Replace the palatal flap and mould it into the vault using firm digital pressure or a warm saline pack for a few minutes to eliminate as much dead space beneath the flap as possible.
8. Place interdental sutures, taking deep bites of the palatal tissue and tying the knot on the labiobuccal side to avoid tongue irritation.

POTENTIAL SURGICAL COMPLICATIONS

- Damage to adjacent teeth.
- Haematoma under palatal flap – infection.
- Necrosis of palatal flap (rare) – if it occurs the necrosed palatal flap is replaced by granulation tissue and scar.
- Perforation of the floor of the maxillary sinus or nose. Best to leave behind deeply embedded apical root fragments.

Surgical exposure of impacted canine

1. The procedure begins in the same way as surgical extraction except that the tooth is left in situ. Extreme caution must be exercised when removing bone so that the crown is not damaged by the burr or chisel.
2. Once the crown of the tooth is located and enough bone is removed to expose the greatest convexity of the crown, a surgical window is cut out of the mucoperiosteal flap which will lie directly over the exposed crown when the flap is replaced.
   Alternatively, if the crown is palpable then a flap need not be raised. Instead, a direct window is cut out of the overlying mucosa and bone to expose the crown of the tooth beyond its maximum convexity.
3. Over the surgically created window, an antiseptic-soaked ribbon gauze is sutured in place to completely cover the exposed crown with non-resorbable sutures.
4. The gauze packing is left in situ for up to 2 weeks to prevent growth of mucosa over the exposed crown during healing.
5. If orthodontic traction is to be used to assist in the eruption of the exposed canine, then the orthodontic bracket may be cemented to the exposed crown either at the time of the surgical exposure, or after the removal of the gauze packing.

Transplantation of maxillary canine

Transplantation of the maxillary canine has evolved from experiences with the reimplantation of avulsed teeth, which follows similar principles.

TECHNIQUE

1. The canine is carefully extracted in one piece. The root surface of the tooth should not be touched with fingers or instruments as it contains

the periodontal ligament cells that are essential to the success of the transplant.

2. A socket is surgically prepared in the maxillary arch that will easily accommodate the transplanted canine with minimal obstruction to its insertion.

   The extracted canine should only be handled by its crown (Figure 7.7) and stored in moist sterile gauze during preparation of the socket to receive the tooth.

   The time between extraction and implantation of the canine should be kept as short as possible to maintain the survival of as many perio-dontal ligament cells as possible.

3. The tooth is implanted in the socket and its position is adjusted into a proper occlusion; the tooth is relieved of all direct occlusal contacts with opposing teeth.

4. Once the canine is implanted into its new position, interdental sutures are placed to approximate the gingival tissues around the canine.

5. Minimal splinting for 4–6 weeks with light interdental wires or glass ionomer bonding to adjacent teeth will permit small physiological move-ments of the transplanted tooth which are found to be conducive to healing of the periodontal membrane. Patients must be instructed not to eat or directly bite on the transplanted tooth for at least 6 months.

6. Light splinting also allows direct inspection of the tooth with easy access for pulpectomy after 7–14 days and eventually root canal therapy

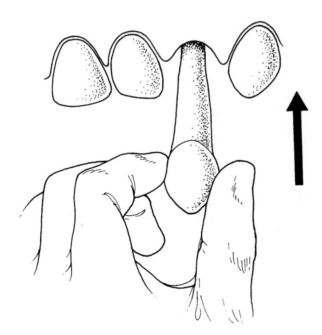

Figure 7.7 Positioning a transplanted maxillary canine in a prepared alveolar socket within the dental arch, holding the tooth only by the crown and not touching the root surface at all.

in 3–6 months, which has been found to eliminate internal root resorption of transplanted teeth in the long term.

PROGNOSIS

The failure rate is approximately 30% over 9 years. Failure is often due to poor surgical technique. Failure with eventual loss of the tooth may arise from:

- Internal root resorption – this has been largely eliminated by the successful application of root canal therapy after transplantation.
- External root resorption – particularly likely when the tooth is forcibly inserted into an inadequately prepared socket.
- Replacement root resorption – where the resorbing root is replaced by bone until the tooth eventually exfoliates.
- Infection – poor aseptic technique, poor oral hygiene and the lack of prophylactic antibiotics may increase the likelihood of infection occurring.

Impacted canines with incomplete root formation have a better success rate than teeth with a closed mature apex owing to the potential for revascularization which eliminates the need for pulpectomy and root canal obturation.

Mandibular second premolars

Causes of impaction

1. Crowded dentition – not enough room in the arch.
2. Potential path of eruption is obstructed by pathology such as a dentigerous cyst, supernumerary tooth, odontoma or odontogenic tumour.
3. Ankylosed mandibular primary molar.

Clinical features

Tooth is often lingually displaced so it may present as:

   a bulge in the lingual alveolus
   erupted or partly erupted through the lingual alveolar plate.

Radiographic investigations

To help localize the tooth the following X-ray films may be useful:

- Lateral mandibular oblique.
- Orthopantomogram.
- Lateral skull.

Treatment options

1. Leave in situ.
2. Extract the awkwardly inclined first premolar to allow the second premolar to erupt into a better position.
3. Orthodontia – to align a lingually displaced second premolar into the arch.
4. Surgical removal.

Surgical removal

Poor access to the lingual alveolus increases the degree of surgical difficulty. It is difficult to raise a lingual flap because the lingual mucosa is very delicate and easily prone to tearing, even with minimal retraction forces. The buccal approach will at least allow better access for instruments to push and luxate the premolar lingually which can then be better grasped.

BUCCAL APPROACH

1. A buccal mucoperiosteal flap is raised.
2. Identify and protect the mental nerve.
3. Remove buccal bone to expose the impacted premolar, taking care to avoid damaging adjacent teeth.
4. Use elevators to luxate and deliver the whole tooth lingually if erupted, or simply divide the tooth and remove the crown and the root separately in the buccal direction if the premolar is unerupted (Figure 7.8).
5. Wound toilet.
6. Close with resorbing sutures.

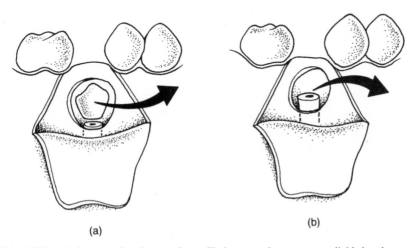

(a)   (b)

Figure 7.8 Surgical approach to impacted mandibular premolars: a, crown divided and removed first; b, remaining root is then subluxated into the space vacated by the removed crown.

Conclusion

Similar surgical principles should be applied when dealing with other impacted teeth such as mandibular canines, incisors, mesiodens or super-numerary teeth. Clinical and radiological assessment, treatment planning and surgical technique for the management of other impacted teeth should all be undertaken in a sensible and logical manner bearing in mind the examples discussed in this chapter.

Further reading

Alling III CC (1993) Management of impacted teeth. *J Oral Maxillofac Surg*, **51** (suppl. 1), 3–6.

Alling III CC, Helfrick JF, Alling RD (1993) *Impacted Teeth*. Philadelphia: Saunders.

Bishara SE (1992) Impacted maxillary canines: a review. *Am J Orthod Dentofac Orthop*, **101**, 159–171.

Edmunds DH, Beck C (1989) Root resorption in autotransplanted maxillary canine teeth. *Int Endo J*, **22**, 19.

Koerner KR, Tilt LV, Johnson KR (1994) *Color Atlas of Minor Oral Surgery*. London: Mosby-Wolfe.

Moore JR, Gillbe GV (1991) *Principles of Oral Surgery*. 4th edn, pp 93–112. Manchester University Press.

Peterson LJ (1992) Rationale for removing impacted teeth: when to extract or not to extract. *J Am Dent Assoc*, **123**, 198–202.

Peterson LJ, Ellis III E, Hupp JR, Tucker MR (1993) *Contemporary Oral and Maxillofacial Surgery*. 2nd edn, pp 225–260. St Louis: Mosby.

Raghoerbar GM, Boering G, Vissink A, Stegenge B (1991) Eruption disturbances of perma-nent molars: a review. *J Oral Pathol Med*, **20**, 159–166.

Tetsch P, Wagner W (1985) *Operative Extraction of Wisdom Teeth*. London: Wolfe.

Zeitler DL (1993) Management of impacted teeth other than third molars. *Oral Maxillofac Surg Clinics North Am*, **5**, 95–103.

8 Odontogenic infections

The surgical management of odontogenic infections is an important part of everyday dental practice. In many instances, antibiotic therapy is only an adjunctive measure to local surgical debridement and drainage of infected tissues. The aim of this chapter is to review the basic principles of anti-microbial therapy and to introduce the surgical protocol for the management of odontogenic infections.

Terminology

Infection – introduction of pathogenic micro-organisms into host tissues that are normally free of the pathogenic micro-organisms. This may lead to tissue destruction as a result of the host inflammatory response to, and the toxic products released by, the invading pathogens.
Odontogenic – arising from the teeth.
Abscess – localized area of inflammation containing pus.
Cellulitis – diffuse inflammation which spreads through soft tissue spaces and along fascial planes, usually as a result of a focus of infection such as an abscess.

Factors determining the extent of infection

Microbe

- Virulence.
- Dose – numbers of infecting microbes.
- Portal of entry – pulp, periodontal tissues, surgical wounds.
- Toxic factors produced and released by infecting microbes.

Host

- **General factors:**
    health status of the patient
    competency of the immune system
    extremes of age – newborn or frail elderly are highly susceptible.
- **Local factors:**
    local blood supply – the greater the vascularity, the better and more effective the host defence systems

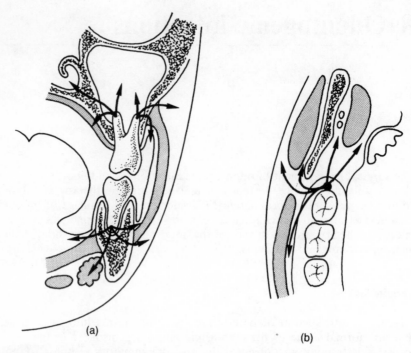

(a)   (b)

Figure 8.1 Anatomical pathways of spread: a, coronal section of oral cavity illustrating the potential pathways of spread of odontogenic infection from the apices of a maxillary and mandibular molar; b, spread of odontogenic infection arising from a mandibular third molar (after Howe).

local anatomy – infection tends to spread along pathways of least resistance such as fascial planes and potential tissue spaces (Figure 8.1).

Natural history of dental infections

See Figure 8.2.

Anatomical pathways of spread of dental infections

MANDIBULAR TEETH

- **Buccinator** – external to body of mandible:
    below attachment – facial swelling
    above attachment – intraoral swelling.
- **Mylohyoid** – internal to body of mandible:
    below – deep sublingual space
    above – superficial sublingual space
    anteriorly – submental space.
- **Masseter** – external to ramus of mandible:
    in-between – submasseteric space
    laterally – temporal space.

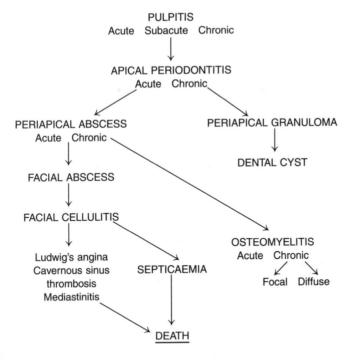

Figure 8.2 Natural history of dental infections.

- **Medial pterygoid** – internal to ramus of mandible:
  laterally – pterygomandibular space
  medially – lateral pharyngeal space
  posteriorly – retropharyngeal space.

MAXILLARY TEETH

- **Buccinator** – laterally:
  above – facial swelling
  below – intraoral swelling.
- **Hard palate** – medially:
  palatal abscess.
- **Maxillary sinus** – superiorly:
  maxillary sinusitis.

Clinical features of dental infections

Local features

1. Pain – toothache.
2. Erythema – gingival inflammation.
3. Oedema – intraoral or facial soft tissue swelling.
4. Pus discharge.
5. Fistula formation.

Systemic features

1. Increased temperature.
2. Increased pulse rate.
3. Increased respiration rate.
4. Lymphadenopathy.
5. Malaise.
6. Increased white blood cell count.

Principles of management of simple dental infections

Local measures

1. Drainage:
     incision into fluctuant swelling (Figures 8.3 and 8.4)
     open root canal
     extract tooth.
2. Maintain drainage:
     insert drainage tube or strip
     warm salt-water mouth rinses.
3. Eliminate the cause:
     extraction of non-vital tooth
     debridement of necrotic tissue
     root canal therapy
     periodontal therapy.

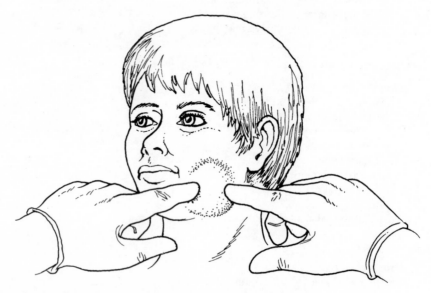

Figure 8.3 Palpating a fluctuant swelling using one finger to press and the other to feel the corresponding movement which may indicate the presence of a fluid-filled tissue space, e.g. an abscess.

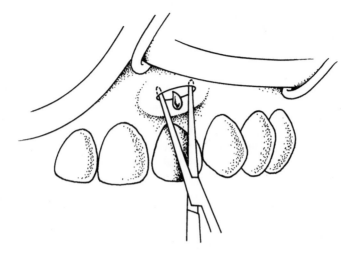

Figure 8.4 Drainage of a dental abscess, using mosquito forceps which are inserted closed through a small incision, then gently opened to establish a larger drainage path for the pus to escape. This is a form of blunt dissection otherwise known as Hilton's method of abscess drainage.

Systemic measures

In conjunction with local measures:

> bed rest and warmth
> maintain adequate fluid intake (administer fluids intravenously if necessary)
> analgesics
> antimicrobial chemotherapy (see below).

Oral infections of surgical significance

Although oral infections may be viral, bacterial, fungal or protozoal, the most common infections of surgical significance are bacterial. In oral surgery practice, the clinician may encounter the following conditions that require surgical attention.

- **Common infections:**
  grossly carious teeth
  periapical abscess or granuloma (see Chapter 9)
  advanced periodontal disease (see Chapter 9)
  pericoronitis.
- **Postoperative infections:**
  dry socket (see Chapter 14)
  buccal space abscess (see Chapter 14)
  infected haematoma (see Chapter 14)
  wound dehiscence and breakdown (see Chapter 14).

- **Uncommon infections:**
    cervicofacial actinomycosis
    osteomyelitis
    Ludwig's angina
    cavernous sinus thrombosis
    mediastinitis.

Pericoronitis

Pericoronitis is inflammation of soft tissue surrounding the crown of a partially erupted tooth. Especially prevalent in lower third molars, recurrent pericoronitis is the most common reason for the extraction of these teeth (see Chapter 6).

AETIOLOGY

The aetiology is unclear – acute episodes usually coincide with stressful periods such as examinations.

PATHOGENESIS

The condition is caused by plaque and food debris collecting under the operculum, which is difficult to clean because of poor access.
    Traumatic occlusion from erupted opposing maxillary third molar may exacerbate the problem.
    Obligate anaerobic bacteria are usually involved.

CLINICAL PRESENTATION

The condition is frequently unilateral.

- **Acute pericoronitis:**
    intermittent severe throbbing pain
    trismus with difficulty eating and swallowing
    swollen and tender operculum with discharging pus
    submandibular lymphadenopathy.
- **Subacute pericoronitis:**
    operculum is less inflamed with little discharge
    continuous dull ache
    pronounced systemic features – increased temperature, pulse and respiration rate, and tender submandibular nodes.
- **Chronic pericoronitis:**
    dull ache which recurs periodically
    radiographs show crater-like radiolucency
    paradental cyst formation.

TREATMENT

1. Gentle saline irrigation under operculum.
2. Caustic solution to establish path of drainage (popular in the past, but seldom used these days).

3. Extract opposing maxillary third molar.
4. Operculectomy contraindicated in the absence of room for the tooth to erupt.
5. Advise patient to use warm salt-water mouth rinses.
6. Analgesics.
7. Antibiotics – where there are systemic signs present, e.g. tender nodes.
8. Extract offending tooth once acute infection has subsided.

Cervicofacial actinomycosis

Subacute or chronic granulomatous infection of the soft tissues of the neck and submandibular region.

PATHOGENESIS

The disease is caused by endogenous commensal oral bacteria such as *Actinomyces israelii, A. viscosus, A. naeslundii* and *A. bovis.*

The histological appearance is of yellow 'sulphur granules' in green pus with tangled masses of gram-positive filaments of actinomycetes surrounded by markedly fibrotic tissue.

Other organisms present are symbiotic and provide anaerobic conditions for actinomycete growth as well as reducing host and local tissue resistance.

CLINICAL PRESENTATION

- **Common lesions:**
    painful periapical abscess in molar or premolar teeth
    associated extensive soft tissue swelling of less than 1 month duration.

TREATMENT

- **Common lesions:**
    drainage of abscess
    extraction of tooth or root canal therapy
    antibiotics – 10 days.
- **Classic lesions:**
    history of surgical trauma (extraction of lower third molar), or mandibular fracture
    chronic soft tissue cervical swelling for more than 3 months
    swelling gradually softens through suppurative necrosis and eventually leads to multiple draining sinuses which yield yellow sulphur granules.
- **Classic lesions:**
    incision and drainage
    antibiotics – a 3–6 week course of either penicillin or tetracycline.

Osteomyelitis

Osteomyelitis is an uncommon inflammatory condition of bone which begins as an infection of the medullary cavity of the jaws and extends to involve the periosteum.

AETIOLOGY

1. Odontogenic infections.
2. Compound jaw fracture.
3. Haematogenous spread from distant site.

PREDISPOSING FACTORS

A compromised blood supply to the bone is a critical factor, with the mandible much more likely to be afflicted than the more vascular maxilla.

- **Local factors:**
    radiotherapy
    vascular thrombosis
    bone disorders, e.g. Paget's disease, osteopetrosis, etc.
- **Systemic factors:**
    malnutrition
    alcoholism
    severe anaemia or sickle cell disease
    leukaemia
    diabetes.

PATHOLOGY

Bone infection results in inflammation followed by tissue necrosis which is compounded by a compromised blood supply. Pus formed in the medullary cavity obstructs the blood supply and so the infected bone becomes necrotic.

The sequestrum (fragment of necrotic bone) is surrounded by an involucrum (reactive new bone formation) (Figure 8.5).

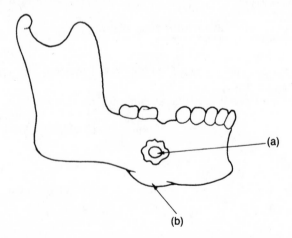

Figure 8.5 Osteomyelitis of the mandible: a, sequestrum – the focus of the infected bone; b, involucrum – reactive new bone formation attempting to establish a border of bone around the destructive focus.

CLASSIFICATION

There are many classifications of osteomyelitis; the simplest is as follows:

1. Suppurative osteomyelitis (pus-forming):
   acute
   chronic – primary or secondary.
2. Non-suppurative osteomyelitis:
   infantile (Garré's)
   chronic sclerosing – focal or diffuse.

Note: osteoradionecrosis is a triad of hypoxia, hypocellularity and hypo-vascularity, and is not primarily an osteomyelitis although the affected bone can become superficially and secondarily infected.

MICROBIOLOGY

Although *Staphylococcus aureus* accounts for half the cases of osteomyelitis in long bones, it is only occasionally found in osteomyelitis of the jaws, particularly where there is an infected extraoral wound.

Organisms that may be isolated from jaw osteomyelitis include anaerobes such as *Bacteroides*, *Fusobacterium* and *Actinomyces*, and other bacteria such as *Klebsiella*, *Pseudomonas* and *Proteus*.

For all cases of osteomyelitis it is essential to send tissue specimens for microbiological culture and antibiotic sensitivity tests.

CLINICAL PRESENTATION

An osteomyelitis of the jaws can present with a varying degree of features ranging from very subtle signs and symptoms to dramatic swelling and intense pain, depending on the type and duration of the disease. A patient with osteomyelitis of the jaws may present with one or more of the following features:

1. Deep, intense pain.
2. Fever, malaise and anorexia.
3. Paraesthesia or anaesthesia of the mental nerve.
4. Loose teeth which may be sensitive to percussion.
5. Firm cellulitis of surrounding soft tissues.
6. Regional lymphadenitis.
7. Fistula formation and pus drainage.
8. Radiological features:
      moth-eaten appearance of bone with zone of radiolucency surrounding sequestrum in advanced stages
      in early stages plain radiographs usually fail to show anything significant; a radioisotope bone scan may be useful to demonstrate areas of increased bone activity where osteomyelitis is suspected.

TREATMENT

- Surgical management – usually undertaken by a specialist oral and maxillofacial surgeon, often in hospital. Surgery involves drainage of pus and removal or resection of necrotic bone.
- Adjunctive therapy – in addition to surgery, patient care is supplemented with:
   fluid and nutritional support
   antibiotic chemotherapy – commenced IV in hospital then changed to oral intake when patient is discharged
   rehabilitation – restoration of jaw function through bone grafting and the provision of a dental prosthesis.

Principles of management of severe infections

Surgical principles

1. Surgical therapy of fascial space infections depends on adequate, open and dependent drainage.
2. Large surgical incisions are necessary to obtain adequate exposure of deep compartments.
3. Communications between fascial planes allows infection to spread readily from one space to another.
4. Secondary spaces as well as primary ones must be drained.
5. Infection and gross swelling may distort the normal anatomy of the face and neck.
6. Repeated surgical drainage and debridement of necrotic tissue may be required.
7. High doses of antibiotics required (IV route preferred) since the poor vascularity of the fascial spaces limits the diffusion of antibiotics into the infected region.

Types of severe infection

In dental practice severe life-threatening infections are uncommon. Although severe infections are managed by specialist units, dentists must be able to recognize the clinical features of the following classic complications that may arise form a dental source, as prompt recognition and referral is a life-saving step.

LUDWIG'S ANGINA

Acute severe bilateral cellulitis of the submandibular and sublingual spaces, often resulting from a primary dental infection of the mandibular second and third molars or after extraction of these teeth.

Presents as a hard, diffuse swelling of the floor of the mouth and neck with a raised tongue, swallowing difficulty, laryngeal oedema and stridor. Airway obstruction is the biggest danger and can lead to death.

Emergency treatment in a specialist hospital unit involves securing an adequate airway, surgical drainage and extraction of offending teeth with parenterally administered high doses of antibiotics, fluids and nutritional support.

CAVERNOUS SINUS THROMBOSIS

Ascending infection arising from the maxillary teeth travels via valveless anterior and posterior facial veins towards the brain.

Presents clinically with exophthalmos, oedema of eyelids, ophthalmo-plegia (paresis of cranial nerves III, IV and VI) and pain, fever and head-ache. If untreated will eventually lead to meningitis and encephalitis with a high mortality.

Neurosurgical management is essential.

MEDIASTINITIS

Although rarely of odontogenic origin, mediastinitis may result from a dental infection which spreads directly along the perivascular space of the carotid sheath into the mediastinum. Can be fatal if treatment is delayed.

Prompt referral to a thoracic surgeon is crucial.

Antibiotics in minor oral surgery

Antibiotic drugs have an important role in the practice of minor oral surgery. The dentist must be fully conversant with the common types of antibiotics used in clinical practice. Because of the potential for drug resistance developing with the indiscriminate use of antibiotics, dentists must be selective as to which antibiotics are prescribed. The indications, drug selection, timing and dosages must be carefully considered in the light of established clinical protocols.

Indications for antibiotics

TREATMENT OF ESTABLISHED INFECTIONS

1. Infections which persist in spite of local measures.
2. Where there are signs of systemic involvement, e.g. submandibular lymphadenopathy or fever.
3. Where surgical access is difficult, e.g. severe trismus.
4. Where there is a diffuse spreading infection (facial cellulitis).

PROPHYLAXIS AGAINST INFECTION

1. Immunocompromised patients.
2. Where the consequences of infection are serious:
    infective endocarditis
    orthopaedic joint prosthesis.

3. Surgical procedures with high likelihood of infection:
   maxillofacial trauma
   major or difficult elective surgery.

Principles of antibiotic use

When prescribing antibiotic therapy, four fundamental considerations need to be addressed.

SELECTION

The type of antibiotic used will depend on the sensitivity of the pathogenic microbe to the antibiotic; this can be decided by:

* Empirical approach – knowing that most dental infections are caused by oral streptococci, most of which are still sensitive to penicillin.
* Scientific approach – taking a specimen of tissue and performing micro-biological cultures and antibiotic sensitivity tests to determine the type of organisms involved and their sensitivity to the various antibiotics.

Note: although more accurate, the scientific approach creates undesirable delays in the institution of antibiotic therapy. In clinical practice this is overcome by commencing empirical therapy until the results of the microbiological tests become available.

CONTACT

Antibiotics cannot diffuse through thick-walled abscesses or into poorly vascularized areas, particularly where necrotic tissues are present. Therefore, to increase the effectiveness of the antibiotic, pus should be drained and necrotic tissues removed wherever possible.

CONCENTRATION

To enhance the effectiveness of the antibiotic, it must be given at regular intervals and in doses that are sufficient to maintain the minimum blood concentration necessary to eliminate all the offending pathogens. Effective blood levels can be rapidly achieved through the intravenous administration of antibiotics, particularly when dealing with severe infections.

TIME

Acute dental infections require 5 days of antibiotic therapy. Chronic low-grade infections (such as actinomycosis) may require up to 6 weeks of antibiotic therapy.

Antibiotics used in minor oral surgery

The most commonly used antibiotics in minor oral surgery practice are the penicillins, erythromycin and metronidazole.

PENICILLINS

Penicillin still remains the first drug of choice in the management of odontogenic infections. It is part of the beta-lactam family of antibiotics which destroy bacteria by interfering with cell wall synthesis. The different penicillins are characterized by the spectrum of activity, the route of administration and their resistance to beta-lactamase-producing bacteria.

- **Spectrum of activity:**
    narrow – e.g. phenoxymethylpenicillin (penicillin V), flucloxacillin
    broad – e.g. amoxycillin, ampicillin, carbenicillin.
- **Route of administration:**
    oral – e.g. phenoxymethylpenicillin (penicillin V), amoxycillin, flucloxacillin
    parenteral (intramuscular or intravenous) – e.g. benzylpenicillin, procaine penicillin, ampicillin, methicillin.
- **Resistance to beta-lactamase-producing bacteria:**
    amoxycillin + clavulanic acid (Augmentin)
    cloxacillin, flucloxacillin, methicillin.

ERYTHROMYCIN

Erythromycin is commonly used as an alternative antibiotic in non-serious odontogenic infections in patients who are allergic to penicillin. It is a narrow-spectrum bacteriostatic antibiotic belonging to the macrolide family of drugs which inhibit bacterial protein synthesis. Erythromycin comes in four types:

1. Base – the active form of erythromycin; it must be coated when administered orally.
2. Stearate – metabolized into the active base before absorption.
3. Estolate – metabolized in the liver into the active base.
4. Lactobionate – parenteral version of erythromycin which is less irritating to veins.

METRONIDAZOLE

Metronidazole is becoming popular as an alternative first drug of choice for odontogenic infections, particularly in Great Britain. It is derived from the imidazole family of drugs which are also used for protozoal, viral and fungal infections. Metronidazole is thought to work by inducing strand breakage of bacterial DNA; however, it is only active against anaerobic micro-organisms.

LESS COMMONLY USED ANTIBIOTICS

There are occasions where the dentist may be faced with the need to prescribe antibiotics that are not normally used in routine practice.

- **Cephalosporins** – Although in the same family of drugs as the penicillins, cephalosporins are seldom used in minor oral surgery since the spectrum, although broad, does not coincide with the predominant bacteria isolated from most odontogenic infections. There is also a 10% cross-allergy with cephalosporins in patients allergic to penicillin.

- **Clindamycin** – a macrolide antibiotic that has become popular for use in serious odontogenic infections in the USA. It is gradually gaining recognition as a more effective alternative to erythromycin in penicillin-sensitive patients.
- **Tetracycline** – its once popular use has declined over the years owing to the increase in resistant organisms associated with odontogenic infections. In spite of this, it is still used for periodontal disease and other chronic infections such as actinomycosis.
- **Other antibiotics** – gentamicin and vancomycin in minor oral surgery practice are confined to prophylactic use in high-risk endocarditis patients admitted to hospital.

Clinical use of antibiotics

In minor oral surgery, antibiotics may be prescribed prophylactically to prevent or minimize surgical infection, or they may be prescribed therapeutically to treat an existing infection.

PROPHYLACTIC USE

For antibiotic prophylaxis in medically compromised patients, see Chapter 15. Indiscriminate use of prophylactic antibiotics for surgical procedures in healthy patients has favoured the survival and increase of drug-resistant bacteria and should therefore not be condoned. Minor oral surgery has a low infection rate in healthy individuals and studies have found no convincing evidence of any benefit from prophylactic antibiotics except where there is overt infection preoperatively. Prophylactic use of antibiotics should therefore comply with the following important principles.

- The surgical procedure should harbour a significant risk for infection, for example:
    long (>30 minutes) or difficult surgery involving significant tissue trauma
    where there is existing infection in and around the surgical site.
- Administration of the antibiotic must be immediately prior to or within 3 hours after the start of surgery:
    the ability of systemic antibiotics to prevent the development of a primary bacterial lesion is confined to the first 3 hours after inoculation of the wound
    commencing prophylactic antibiotic cover the day before surgery only leads to the development of resistant organisms
    continuing antibiotics for days after the surgery has not been shown to decrease the incidence of wound infection.
- Prophylactic antibiotics should be given at twice the usual dose over the shortest effective time so as to minimize the potential side-effects of long-term use (e.g. diarrhoea) and prevent the growth of resistant bacteria.

- There are many antibiotic prophylactic regimens currently used so the following examples are just a few that may be considered:
    amoxycillin 3 g orally, 45 minutes before surgery under local anaesthesia
    clindamycin 600 mg orally, 30 minutes before surgery under LA for penicillin-sensitive patients
    benzylpenicillin 600 mg IM/IV on induction for procedures under general anaesthesia
    erythromycin lactobionate 500 mg IV on induction for GA procedures in patients allergic to penicillin.

Note: the last two regimens may be followed with an additional oral dose 6 hours after the initial dose.

THERAPEUTIC USE

For the effective treatment of odontogenic infections, antibiotic therapy is best used as an adjunctive measure to surgical drainage and debridement wherever possible. Where facilities are available, pus or tissue specimens should always be sent for microbiological analysis and antibiotic sensitivity tests. While the microbiological assessment is being carried out, the patient should commence an empirical antibiotic regimen until the results are available, when the antibiotics may be changed in light of the microbial sensitivity data obtained. Suggested empirical regimens are as follows:

- **Mild odontogenic infections:**
    penicillin V orally, 500 mg first dose then 250 mg four times daily 1 hour before meals (5 day course)
    erythromycin orally, 500 mg first dose then 250 mg four times daily for 5 days in patients allergic to penicillin.
- **Moderate odontogenic infections:**
    amoxycillin 500 mg orally three times daily for 5–7 days; may need to add metronidazole 400 mg orally three times daily for 7 days
    clindamycin orally, 300 mg first dose then 150–300 mg four times daily for 5–7 days for patients allergic to penicillin.
- **Severe odontogenic infection** (must be treated in hospital):
    benzylpenicillin IV 1.2 g first dose then 600 mg every 6 hours with metronidazole IV 500 mg every 8 hours for a few days until acute episode subsides sufficiently for the patient to continue safely with an oral regimen
    clindamycin IV 600 mg first dose then 300 mg IV every 6 hours for penicillin-sensitive patients
    may need to add gentamicin 80 mg IV every 8 hours, but monitor blood levels if drug is given for more than 36 hours.

Side-effects of antibiotics

It is the responsibility of the clinician prescribing the medication to warn the patient about the potential side-effects of antibiotic drugs. The most common side-effects are as follows.

- **Penicillins:**
  hypersensitivity in 2–8% of the population; severe anaphylaxis is more likely to occur with IV administration
  vaginal thrush in some women
  inactivation of the female contraceptive pill (especially ampicillin and amoxycillin)
  safe in pregnancy and lactation.
- **Erythromycin:**
  gastric irritation – nausea and vomiting
  the estolate type may cause intrahepatic cholestatic jaundice in pregnant women.
- **Metronidazole:**
  oral candidal overgrowth – tongue discolouration
  darkening of urine
  avoid with alcohol (causes vomiting)
  avoid in pregnancy – theoretical carcinogenic data in animals.
- **Clindamycin:**
  severe diarrhoea – pseudomembranous colitis (treated with metronidazole).
- **Tetracycline:**
  staining and malformation of bones and teeth during formative years – drug contraindicated in pregnancy and children less than 8 years old
  diarrhoea – floral imbalance
  superinfection – candidal overgrowth.

Further reading

Bridgeman A, Wiesenfeld D, Hellyar A, Sheldon W (1995) Major maxillofacial infections. An evaluation of 107 cases. *Aust Dent J*, **40**, 281–288.

Flynn TR (1991) Odontogenic infections. In *Infections of the Head and Neck* (DM Laskin, RA Strauss, eds). *Oral Maxillofac Surg Clinics North Am*, **3**, 311–330.

Haug RH, Hoffman MJ, Indresano AT (1991) An epidemiological and anatomic survey of odontogenic infections. *J Oral Maxillofac Surg*, **49**, 976–980.

Indresano AT, Haug RH, Hoffman MJ (1992) The third molar as a cause of deep space infections. *J Oral Maxillofac Surg*, **50**, 33.

Marsh P, Martin M (1992) *Oral Microbiology*. 3rd edn. London: Chapman & Hall.

Peterson LJ (1990) Antibiotic prophylaxis against wound infections in oral and maxillofacial surgery. *J Oral Maxillofac Surg*, **48**, 617.

Pogrel MA (1993) Infection management. In *Dentoalveolar surgery* (CC Alling III, ed.). *Oral Maxillofac Surg Clinics North Am*, **5**, 127–136.

Topazian RG, Goldberg MH, eds (1987) *Oral and Maxillofacial Infections*. 2nd edn. Philadelphia: Saunders.

Walton JG, Thompson JW, Seymour RA (1994) *Textbook of Dental Pharmacology and Therapeutics*. 2nd edn. Oxford University Press.

9 Surgical conservation of teeth

Surgery may be used to conserve teeth that would otherwise be destined for extraction. Specialists in endodontics and periodontics occasionally resort to surgery as a means of helping to retain teeth with advanced disease that cannot be adequately treated with conventional restorative therapy alone. The aim of this chapter is to present a broad outline of surgical techniques that are used to prolong the useful life of teeth afflicted with advanced periodontal and endodontic lesions.

Terminology

Endodontics – a branch of dentistry that deals with the diagnosis and management of diseases of the dental pulp and associated structures.
Periodontics – a branch of dentistry that deals with the diagnosis and management of diseases of the periodontium and associated supporting structures of the dental apparatus.

Endodontic surgery

Once the realm of oral surgery practice, endodontic surgery has become an important part of specialist endodontic practice. Where the root canal system of the tooth cannot be thoroughly debrided or properly obturated, surgical endodontics offers the only practical alternative to extraction of the tooth.

Indications for endodontic surgery

- Failure of non-surgical treatment – where non-surgical treatment is impossible (e.g. non-negotiable complex apical canal system) or ineffective (e.g. persistent symptoms) in resolving a canal or periapical problem.
- Persistent pain – not adequately relieved by pulp extirpation.
- Establishing drainage – of a symptomatic periapical radiolucent area of infection above the tooth that cannot be drained through its canal.
- Procedural problems such as root perforation, instrument breakage or apical damage due to overzealous root canal therapy.
- Biopsy – periapical tissue specimens may be required for histological diagnosis, particularly where the associated tooth is vital.

- Patient convenience – combining root canal therapy and apical surgery in one visit is possible and within the acceptable standards of patient care provided the single visit is requested by the patient.

Surgical procedures

Endodontic surgery is always accompanied by pulp extirpation, root canal debridement and obturation, either prior to surgery – which is more acceptable – or at the same time as surgery – where adequate sterility is difficult to achieve.

Endodontic surgery encompasses the following procedures.

PERIAPICAL SURGERY

Periapical surgery deals with the surgical management of pathology surrounding the apices of teeth. Procedures may include drainage, biopsy curettage or enucleation of lesions in a region of alveolar bone around the apical third of a root.

APICECTOMY

Apicectomy is the partial or complete resection of the apical third segment of the root of a tooth. Often, this procedure is accompanied by the insertion of a retrograde root filling to seal the exposed apical portion of the canal.

ROOT AMPUTATION AND HEMISECTION

A salvage technique used for multirooted teeth (e.g. molars) where the non-restorable root is surgically removed in order to improve the prognosis of the remaining tooth. Hemisection is where part of the crown is also removed together with the non-restorable root.

Surgical technique

FLAP DESIGN

There are two types of flap design (Figure 9.1):

- Flaps that do not involve the gingival margin:
  semilunar
  modified scalloped semilunar.
- Flaps that involve the gingival margins:
  gingival
  triangular
  trapezoidal.

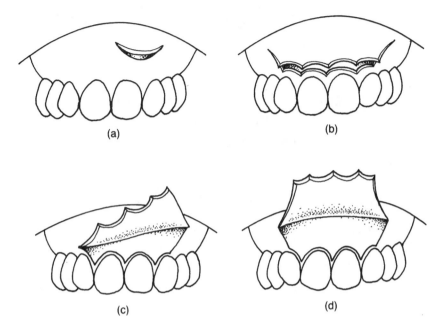

Figure 9.1 Endodontic flap design: a, semilunar; b, modified scalloped semilunar; c, triangular gingival; d, trapezoidal gingival.

BONE REMOVAL

A round surgical burr is used to make a cortical bony window exposing the periapical region and root surface of the tooth. The incision outline of the flap *must* always rest on sound bone at the end of the operation.

OPERATIVE PROCEDURES

Once the desired exposure is achieved the clinician may perform any one of the following procedures:

- Drainage of a periapical abscess.
- Curettage of a periapical granuloma.
- Enucleation of a dental (radicular) cyst.
- Apicectomy with retrograde root filling (Figure 9.2). It is best to bevel the apicectomy towards the facial aspect for better visibility and access to the exposed apical canal. The choice of retrograde filling is a matter of personal preference although amalgam still appears to be popular.
- Surgical amputation of a root – requires a much wider surgical access.
- Hemisection – surgical removal of a root and part of the crown.

CLOSURE

Immediately prior to closure the clinician must consider the following important steps:

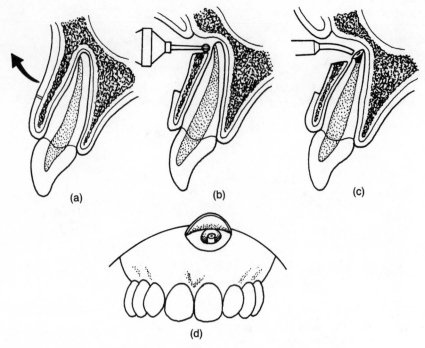

Figure 9.2 Apicectomy technique: a, raising a labial flap; b, round burr used to remove buccal bone to surgically expose apex of tooth; c, apicectomy with retrograde seal being placed in prepared apical root; d, frontal view demonstrating the angulation of the apicectomized surface of the root apex facing labially for easier access.

1. Wound toilet – removal of loose bits of tooth, bone, filling material and other small debris and thorough irrigation of surgical site.
2. Complete haemostasis – bleeding surgical site may be packed with simple gauze under finger pressure for 5–10 minutes or local haemostatic agents may be used such as fibrillar collagen, bone wax, Gelfoam or Surgicel.
3. Periapical X-rays – where a root filling has been undertaken, either ortho- or retrograde or both, then a periapical radiograph must be taken, developed and checked prior to final closure of wound.
4. Suturing – suture type and technique is a matter of personal preference although 4/0 tends to be the most popular size.

Anatomical considerations

The complexity of endodontic surgery is essentially dictated by access to the apical root and the surrounding anatomy of the region.

ACCESS

1. Incisors and canines have a simple root morphology and by virtue of their anterior position in the mouth, the apices of these teeth are readily accessible.

2. Posterior teeth – accessibility is much more restricted, particularly with the palatal roots of the maxillary premolars and molars.

SURROUNDING ANATOMY

1. Maxillary premolars and first molars – the apices are often found to penetrate the floor of the maxillary sinus, therefore increasing the likelihood of a direct breach of the maxillary sinus and a supervening sinusitis occurring.
2. Mandibular premolars and molars – the close proximity of the inferior alveolar and mental nerve to the apices of these teeth increases the likelihood of nerve damage resulting from endodontic surgical procedures with impairment of lower lip sensation.

Periodontal surgery

Periodontal disease is a common affliction in any adult population and, as such, deserves a great deal more attention than is commonly given in general dental practice. Unlike endodontic surgery which is used to *eliminate* a disease process, the aim of periodontal surgery is to *contain* a disease process in order to improve the longevity of a tooth or teeth.

Indications for periodontal surgery

Periodontal surgery is often used as a last resort to treat advanced periodontal disease that has failed to respond adequately to more conservative measures such as scaling and root planing.

Surgical periodontal disease

Periodontal lesions that are amenable to surgery may be broadly classified into three groups:

1. Suprabony pockets – the simplest of lesions where the epithelial attachment has migrated apically along the root surface to create periodontal pockets that are totally surrounded by soft tissues.
2. Infrabony pockets – where the base of the pocket has progressed apically to the crest of the alveolar bone so that one or more of the pocket walls are bounded by bone.
3. Complicated pockets – periodontal pockets that are complicated by mucogingival problems such as high muscle attachments or the absence of attached gingiva.

Aims of periodontal surgery

Periodontal surgery is used to achieve the following goals:

• Pocket elimination or reduction – by surgically removing or reducing soft tissues that would otherwise promote plaque accumulation and hinder simple hygiene measures.

- Promoting reattachment – in some cases where root exposure is un-desirable (e.g. maxillary incisors) a more conservative surgical approach may be used, where rather than eliminating the periodontal pocket, the flap is replaced in its original position. The long junctional epithelium thus produced is inherently unstable and demands higher standards of plaque control than for pocket elimination procedures.
- Bone reshaping – so that after healing and remodelling the resultant alveolar architecture will permit effective oral hygiene measures to be carried out.
- Guided tissue regeneration (GTR) – the science of guided tissue regen-eration using flexible Teflon membranes (e.g. Gortex) or barriers that prevent the ingrowth of undesirable cells during the healing phase, may help promote the regeneration of periodontal ligament cells and new bone in advanced periodontal disease.
- Correction of mucogingival problems – which result in lack of attached gingiva; may be caused by:
  periodontal pocketing or gingival recession
  pull on the gingival margin (e.g. high fraenum)
  shallow vestibular sulcus depth.

Periodontal surgical techniques

Periodontal surgery is a vast subject in its own right and it would be beyond the scope of this small book to describe each procedure in detail. A simple introduction to the various procedures is given to enable the reader to develop some idea of the scope of periodontal surgery. A reading list for more detailed perusal is provided at the end of this chapter.

GINGIVECTOMY

Gingivectomy is performed where more conservative periodontal proce-dures cannot eliminate suprabony pockets larger than 4 mm or persistent gingival swelling with false pocket formation. There are two types of gingi-vectomy procedures (Figure 9.3).

- **Classic technique** – the complete removal of the gingival soft tissue wall of a periodontal pocket leaving an open wound with an adequate zone of attached gingiva which is left to heal by secondary intention.
- **Inverse bevel gingivectomy** – a flap procedure which allows access for the treatment of underlying bone defects and direct primary closure of wound, although not as much gingival soft tissue is removed as in the classic technique.

FLAP PROCEDURES

Flap procedures have the advantages of allowing access to the root and alveolar bone, less tissue sacrifice, primary closure and improved tissue morphology after healing. The different flap procedures are used for speci-fic problems as outlined below.

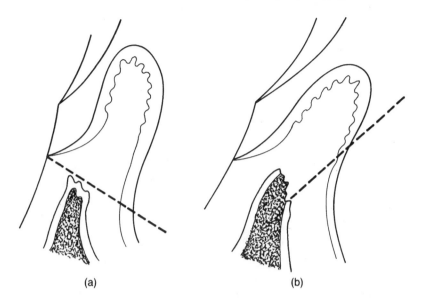

(a)   (b)

Figure 9.3 Gingivectomy incisions: a, classic bevel incision; b, inverse bevel incision.

- **Inverse bevel gingivectomy** – used for pocket elimination or reduction by the removal of gingival soft tissues (see above).
- **Apically repositioned flap** – used for pocket elimination or reduction by moving the flap in an apical direction (Figure 9.4).
- **Modified Widman flap** – used as a technique for open curettage aimed at reattachment rather than pocket elimination. More conservative than pocket elimination procedures as it involves replacing the flap in its original position to avoid root exposure.
- **Laterally repositioned flap** – where a full thickness gingival flap is raised and rotated to cover a localized defect of a single adjacent tooth. The defect may have significant recession of the gingival margin with considerable exposure of the root which is often associated with an underlying bone dehiscence. The donor site is left to heal by secondary intention (Figure 9.5).
- **Coronally repositioned flap** – used in conjunction with a free gingival graft, a mucoperiosteal flap containing the healed gingival graft is raised and positioned coronally to cover the exposed root surfaces of the teeth. It has only limited success, with postoperative shrinkage and pocket recurrence a likely outcome.

OSTEOPLASTY/OSTECTOMY

With the aid of flap procedures, direct access to alveolar bone is established for osteoplasty (bone shaping) and ostectomy (bone removal) for the purpose of obtaining an acceptable bone shape that is more amenable to cleaning.

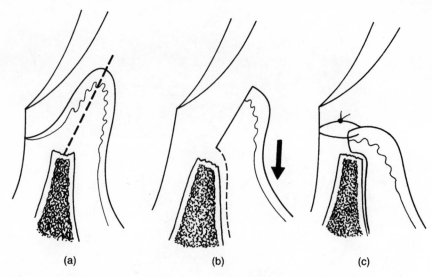

Figure 9.4 Apically repositioned flap: a, crevicular incision; b, gingival flap repositioned in the apical direction; c, gingival margin fixed in new apical position with sutures.

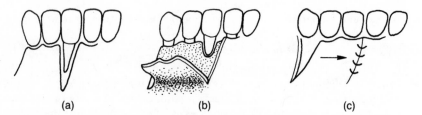

Figure 9.5 Laterally positioned flap: a, dehiscence of incisor with outline of flap incision; b, mucoperiosteal flap raised; c, flap transposed laterally to cover dehiscence leaving a secondary defect that will heal by secondary intention.

GUIDED TISSUE REGENERATION

New bone or periodontal ligament formation may be achieved in a defect by removing the surrounding inflamed tissues and inserting a temporary flexible Teflon membrane over the surgical site to prevent ingrowth of rapidly proliferating fibrous connective tissue. The membrane will act as a barrier that will promote the development of the slower-growing desirable cells required for bone and periodontal ligament regeneration (Figure 9.6).

FREE GRAFTS

In periodontal surgery, there is an occasional need to use free tissue grafts to provide additional tissue in areas of deficiency. There are two types of grafts which may be used:

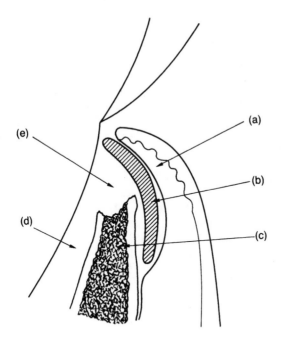

Figure 9.6 Guided tissue regeneration: a, margin of gingival flap; b, flexible Teflon membrane; c, eroded alveolar bone margin; d, periodontal membrane; e, space where new bone and periodontal membrane is expected to develop under the protection of the Teflon membrane.

- **Free gingival grafts** – a small piece of keratinized mucosa, usually procured from an edentulous area or the palate, is transplanted to form a new zone of attached gingiva. Particularly useful in areas where the attached gingiva is deficient or destroyed, and where a fraenum or high muscle attachment needs to be surgically repositioned away from the gingival margin, leaving a defect that is suitably repaired by a free gingival graft.
- **Free bone grafts** – used to fill in alveolar bone defects since simple bone curettage is an unpredictable way of stimulating new bone formation. Bone grafts may be autogenous (derived from another site in the same patient), xenogenic (treated animal bone such as bovine mineral apatite) or synthetic (e.g. hydroxyapatite or Perioglass). The use of guided tissue regeneration techniques have enabled a more predictable method of new bone formation.

OTHER TECHNIQUES

Periodontal surgery also includes surgical procedures that are not confined to the management of periodontal disease but may be used in preprosthetic or endodontic surgery.

- **Fraenectomy** – when the fraenum inserts into the gingival margin, movement of the lips and hence the tugging action of the fraenum on the gingiva may result in gingival detachment from the tooth. Gingival inflammation and pocketing may be further aggravated by a high fraenal attachment. The surgical removal of a fraenum via a Z-plasty or diamond excision with primary closure may, on the one hand, solve the mucogingival problem, but on the other hand, may result in the loss of attached gingiva. The loss of attached gingiva is usually managed with a free gingival graft to the area where the fraenum once attached to the gingival margin.
- **Sulcus deepening procedures** – may be used where a shallow sulcus results in a mucogingival problem that is detrimental to periodontal health. The Edlan technique of sulcus deepening involves transposing the labial mucosa with the alveolar periosteum, although this may create tightening of the lower lip.
- **Root resection or hemisection** – also used in endodontic surgery (see above), this procedure is useful in periodontics where extensive bone loss around one of the roots of a multirooted tooth can be managed through the removal of the affected root, thereby improving the prognosis for the rest of the tooth. This procedure requires root canal therapy of the tooth prior to surgery (Figure 9.7).

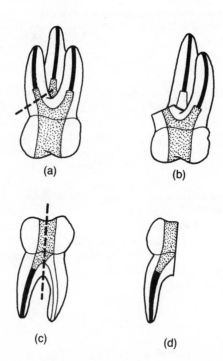

(a)

(b)

(c)

(d)

Figure 9.7 Root resection and hemisection: a, root resection outline; b, resultant tooth after root resection; c, hemisection outline; d, resultant tooth after hemisection.

Adjunctive measures

Although periodontal surgery follows the common basic surgical principles, there are two essential measures that are unique to this specialty.

ROOT SCALING AND PLANING

Particularly where flap procedures are used, root scaling and planing form an essential part of the surgery, without which the main objectives of disease control could not be achieved.

PERIODONTAL DRESSING

After all periodontal surgical procedures, a periodontal dressing is used to cover the wound.

- **Functions of a periodontal dressing:**
  to protect the wound from irritation
  to maintain a clean wound
  to control bleeding
  to provide postoperative comfort
  to promote healing and prevent exuberant scar tissue production.
- **Requirements of a periodontal dressing:**
  non-irritant and non-allergenic
  easily applied and adapted to the teeth and tissues so that it is well retained
  a slow setting time to allow manipulation between the teeth
  antibacterial
  provides adequate seal against food and saliva
  should set fairly hard and not be easily displaced
  acceptable taste.
- **Types of periodontal dressing:**
  Although numerous dressing are based on the zinc oxide–eugenol mixture, some patients may be allergic to eugenol or may find the taste of it unacceptable. Eugenol-free dressings such as Coe-pack and Peripak may overcome these problems.
- **Placement technique:**
  apply the dressing carefully so that it covers the wound and fills the interdental spaces completely
  the dressing should be muscle trimmed by movement of the lips, cheeks and tongue before it sets
  excess dressing, particularly over the occlusal surfaces of the teeth, should be carefully removed
  the dressing is usually removed after 1 week, and the wound completely irrigated with warm water
  a new dressing may need to be applied for a further week if the wound is not sufficiently epithelialized following gingivectomy procedures.

Further reading

Carranza FA (1990) *Clinical Periodontology*. 7th edn. Philadelphia: Saunders.

Genco RJ, Goldman HM, Cohen DW (1990) *Contemporary Periodontics*. St Louis: Mosby.

Gutman JL, Harrison JW (1991) *Surgical Endodontics*. Oxford: Blackwell.

Hoag PM, Powlak EA (1990) *Essentials of Periodontics*. St Louis: Mosby.

Ito T, Johnson JD (1994) *Color Atlas of Periodontal Surgery*. London: Mosby-Wolfe.

Koerner KR, Tilt LV, Johnson KR (1994) *Color Atlas of Minor Oral Surgery*. London: Mosby-Wolfe.

Walton RE, Torabinejad M (1989) *Principles and Practice of Endodontics*. Philadelphia: Saunders.

10 The maxillary sinus

Because of the close anatomical proximity of the maxillary sinus to the oral cavity, the dental surgeon may occasionally come across sinus pathology during minor oral surgical procedures. This is especially likely when sinus disease presents with oral symptoms such as a palatal swelling or tender maxillary teeth. The aim of this chapter is to present an outline of the relationship between maxillary sinus pathology and minor oral surgery.

Terminology

Sinus – unlike the true surgical meaning, 'sinus' in this chapter is used interchangeably with 'antrum' to denote an aerated natural cavity within the facial skeleton lined by respiratory epithelium which communicates with the nasal cavity.
Oroantral communication – an unnatural communication between the oral cavity and maxillary sinus.
Communication or perforation – a communication existing for less than 48 hours.
Fistula – epithelial-lined tract that forms after 48 hours.

Note: in its true meaning a fistula is an abnormal communication between two epithelial lined surfaces.

Anatomy of the maxillary sinus

Description

The maxillary sinus (Figure 10.1) is also known as the antrum of Highmore. It constitutes one of the paranasal sinuses, the others being the frontal, sphenoid and ethmoid sinuses. It arises as an outgrowth of the lining of the embryonic nasal cavity into the surrounding bone that goes on to form the maxilla. The sinus is basically a hollow cavity in each of the two maxillary bones, which is lined by respiratory epithelium (pseudo-stratified ciliated columnar epithelium).

Boundaries

Pyramidal in shape, the maxillary sinus has the following boundaries:

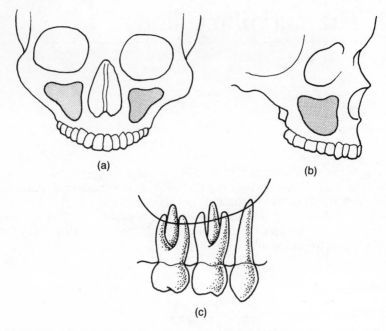

Figure 10.1 Anatomy of the maxillary sinus: a, frontal view; b, lateral view; c, maxillary sinus floor in relation to the roots of the posterior maxillary teeth.

- Base – lateral wall of the nose.
- Apex – projects laterally into the zygomatic process of the maxilla.
- Roof – orbital floor.
- Floor – alveolar process of maxilla which supports the premolars and molars.
- Posterior wall – infratemporal and pterygopalatine fossa.
- Anterior wall – facial surface of maxilla.

Communications

- Drainage – via ostium (hiatus semilunaris) under middle concha of lateral nasal wall.
- Nerve supply – infraorbital nerve (maxillary division of trigeminal V_2 nerve).
- **Blood supply:**
  upper part – anterior ethmoidal artery
  medial wall – sphenopalatine artery
  anterolateral wall – infraorbital artery
  posterolateral wall – posterior superior alveolar artery
  (accompanied by similar veins).
- **Lymphatic drainage:**
  submandibular nodes
  retropharyngeal nodes.

The maxillary sinus and the dental surgeon

There are three instances where the dental surgeon may be involved with the maxillary sinus:

1. Creation of an oroantral communication (OAC).
2. Displacement of a tooth fragment into the sinus.
3. Diagnosis of maxillary sinus pathology.

Oroantral communications

- **Causes of OAC:**
    dental extractions – see 'predisposing factors' below
    facial trauma – particularly gunshot wounds to the midface
    preprosthetic surgery – unintentional complication of bony reduction
    of pneumatized maxillary tuberosity
    osteomyelitis or osteoradionecrosis of maxillary alveolus
    malignant neoplasm eroding through the alveolus.
- **Predisposing factors:**
    roots of maxillary premolars and molars penetrating the sinus floor
    hypercementosis or ankylosis of maxillary premolars and molars
    lone standing maxillary molars, particularly in elderly patients
    bulbous curved roots of maxillary premolars and molars
    traumatic extraction of maxillary posterior teeth
    periapical pathology associated with posterior maxillary teeth
    large maxillary sinus and pneumatized maxillary tuberosity
    neoplasms.
- **Clinical features:**
    nasal regurgitation of liquids
    altered nasal resonance
    cannot suck through straw or cigarette
    unilateral nasal discharge
    bad taste in mouth
    bubbling through OAC when nose is occluded under pressure.

Natural history

If left untreated an OAC may result in the following:

    spontaneous healing – less likely with communications larger than 5 mm
    in diameter
    oroantral fistula formation – an epithelial lined tract that forms about
    48 hours after the creation of the OAC
    acute maxillary sinusitis
    chronic maxillary sinusitis.

Management

When an OAC is created upon extraction of a maxillary premolar or molar, the clinician should confirm its presence by occluding the patient's nose under pressure and watching for bubbling arising from the extraction site.

IMMEDIATE MANAGEMENT

There are four choices (Figure 10.2):

1. Replace the extracted tooth and splint into position with sutures or interdental wiring to adjacent teeth. Arrange for surgical extraction of the tooth in 4–6 weeks.
2. Attempt primary closure by reducing the edge of the bony socket and bringing together the buccal and palatal gingival margins with simple suturing.
3. Insert a dressing pack – for a large OAC a non-resorbable pack or dressing (Bismuth Iodoform Paraffin Paste, ribbon gauze soaked with Whitehead's varnish) may be sutured over the defect and removed after 2 weeks to allow healing by secondary intention.
4. Attempt formal closure by raising a buccal or palatal flap which is advanced or rotated over the defect to completely cover the OAC (see below).

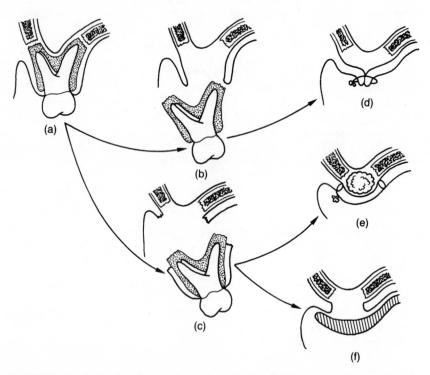

Figure 10.2 Creation by dental extraction and repair of an OAC: a, traumatic extraction of a maxillary first molar; b, tooth removed together with bony floor of maxillary sinus; c, fracture of maxillary sinus floor and tearing of surrounding gingival margin; d, simple closure by direct suture of apposing gingival margins; e, sealing the defect with an antiseptic-soaked pack sutured into position; f, covering the OAC defect with a flange of a prosthesis.

PATIENT INSTRUCTIONS

A patient with an OAC that is either suspected or confirmed should be discharged with the following instructions:

avoid blowing nose – for at least 10 days or up to 3 weeks depending on the size of the defect; simply wipe a running nose
avoid the following – smoking, sucking through straws, blowing up balloons, or playing wind instruments – for at least 10 days.

POSTOPERATIVE MEDICATION

The sinus passages may be irritated by oral flora seeping through the OAC and causing an inflamed and congested antral lining. There is also a high risk of sinus infection. The following medications are recommended to prevent or minimize the likelihood of sinusitis as well as for patient comfort.

Nasal decongestants
Sympathomimetic and antihistamine class of drugs.

- **Local:**
  nasal sprays or nasal drops
  examples: ephedrine sulphate 0.5–1.0% or phenylephrine hydrochloride (Neo-Synephrine)
  may produce rebound effects if used alone for more than 3 days.
- **Systemic:**
  examples: pseudoephedrine (Sudafed) 30–60 mg three times daily or diphenhydramine
  act synergistically with local medication to reduce rebound effects.

Mucolytic agents
To encourage spontaneous easy drainage from sinus.

examples: camphor or menthol dispensed in different inhalant forms.

Antibiotics
A range of antibiotics effective against common upper respiratory tract infections may also be useful in preventing or treating sinusitis. These include:

amoxycillin
co-trimoxazole
erythromycin
tetracycline.

Analgesics
For sinus pain, the most useful oral analgesics are the compound formulas that combine a non-steroidal anti-inflammatory drug with a decongestant, for example paracetamol 500 mg + pseudoephedrine 30 mg.

DELAYED MANAGEMENT

In some situations, formal closure of an OAC may have to be delayed a few weeks to:

allow time for any acute sinus infection to resolve with medication
allow for natural reduction in size of the OAC defect so that subsequent surgery is simplified, i.e. smaller flaps are required for formal closure
allow for the possibility that the OAC may heal spontaneously, thereby eliminating the need for surgical intervention.

SURGICAL REPAIR OF AN OAC

There must be no active sinus infection immediately prior to closure and consideration should be given to the provision of adequate intranasal drainage. Surgical repair should be left to experienced clinicians. There are numerous surgical techniques for closure of an OAC; however, in this chapter only three of the most common procedures are discussed.

Buccal advancement flap
Repair using a buccal advancement flap is the simplest and least morbid procedure, easily performed under local anaesthesia with uniformly excellent results (Figures 10.3 and 10.4).

- **Technique:**
    excision of epithelium around the edges of the OAC or removal of fistulous tract from an oroantral fistula
    raise a triangular mucoperiosteal buccal flap with an extended curvilinear mesial releasing incision
    horizontal incision to release the periosteum at the base of the flap

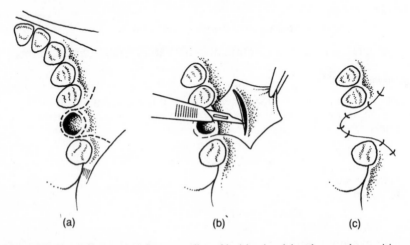

(a)   (b)   (c)

Figure 10.3 Buccal advancement flap: a, outline of incision involving the complete excision of the fistula; b, raising a buccal flap and incising the periosteum to allow advancement of the flap; c, suturing the flap into position.

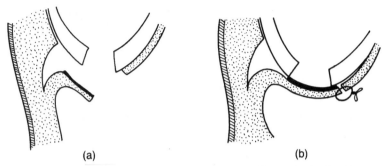

Figure 10.4 Coronal view of buccal flap: a, raising the buccal flap and releasing the periosteum; b, flap placed across the alveolus to cover the defect (after Howe).

advance the buccal flap across the defect so that the edge of the flap lies passively next to the palatal mucosal margin

simple interrupted late-resorbing sutures (e.g. 3/0 Vicryl) used to fix the flap over the defect

there is some reduction in buccal sulcus depth which tends to re-model in 4–8 weeks.

Palatal rotation flap
The palatal rotation flap procedure is difficult to perform in a fully con-scious patient. In spite of the good results, there is a fair degree of morbid-ity involved with this procedure (Figure 10.5).

- **Technique:**
  excision of epithelium around the edges of the OAC or removal of fistulous tract from an oroantral fistula

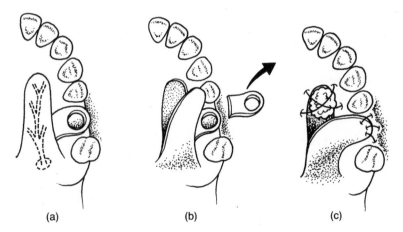

Figure 10.5 Palatal rotation flap: a, outline of incisions with schematic diagram of axial blood supply of the palatal flap by the greater palatine artery; b, raising of palatal flap and excision of fistula; c, rotated palatal flap sutured in position and secondary defect covered with antiseptic-soaked ribbon gauze which is also fixed in position with sutures.

a long palatal finger flap based on the greater palatine artery is raised
and rotated across the arch to cover the defect
ribbon gauze soaked in antiseptic is sutured over the exposed donor
site of palatine bone and left in situ for 3 weeks to heal by secondary
intention
only limited flap rotation is possible because of the danger of kinking
the axial blood supply, thereby creating venous congestion
uneven palatal surface regains normal flat appearance in 2 months.

Buccal fat pad pedicled graft

An ingenious and simple method uses vascularized buccal fat to obturate
the oroantral defect with relatively little morbidity.

- **Technique:**
    excision of epithelium around the edges of the OAC or removal of
    fistulous tract from an oroantral fistula
    horizontal buccal incision in maxillary third molar region
    buccal fat is gently teased out of its cheek bed and advanced into
    the defect either by direct rotation or by tunnelling under the
    mucosa
    the transposed fat pad epithelializes in 2–3 weeks with the attached
    pedicle which provides its nutrients through its arterial supply.

Foreign bodies in the maxillary sinus

Foreign bodies of dental origin

Occasionally, during an extraction or root canal therapy of a maxillary
premolar or molar, a tooth, root fragment or endodontic filling material
may be displaced into the maxillary sinus.

Immediate action

When an object is displaced into the sinus the clinician should take the
following steps:

1. Stop! If you suspect the fragment has been displaced into the sinus, do
   not continue instrumenting the area as you are likely to displace the
   fragment even further into a more inaccessible position.
2. Inform the patient.
3. Radiographic investigations – two radiographs should be taken at right
   angles to each other, e.g. an occipitomental view and a lateral cephalogram. This is used to help determine if the object is lying:
       in the sinus cavity proper
       between the sinus lining and its bony wall
       in the soft tissues outside the maxilla.

Definitive management

FRESH ALVEOLAR WOUND

1. Raise a flap above the tooth in question.
2. Enlarge the socket or create a bony window into the sinus.
3. Localize and remove the fragment with the help of a fine suction tip.
4. Plan flap incisions that will allow direct and complete closure of the OAC.

HEALED ALVEOLAR WOUND

The following procedure is for experienced clinicians only!

1. Use the Caldwell-Luc approach, preferably under general anaesthesia.
2. A 3 cm vestibular incision is made from the upper canine to the second premolar.
3. A mucoperiosteal flap is raised to expose the anterolateral surface of the maxilla.
4. Important structures to avoid damaging:
     apices of canine and premolar teeth
     infraorbital foramen and nerve.
5. A window of bone is removed to reveal the sinus cavity and allowing direct inspection and unobstructed access to the whole maxillary sinus.
6. After location and removal of fragment, the vestibular incision is primarily closed with a continuous suture.

Diagnosis of maxillary sinus pathology

On occasions the dental surgeon may encounter diseases arising from the maxillary sinus that present with oral signs and symptoms. Furthermore, dental radiographs may reveal abnormalities within the maxillary sinus that need further attention or referral for specialist opinion and management. Whatever the circumstances, the dental surgeon must be able to immediately recognize sinus pathology, as prompt referral – particularly in cases of malignant disease – can be life-saving for the patient. Although diseases of the maxillary sinus are commonly managed by ear, nose and throat surgeons, there are cases that can be treated equally well by most oral and maxillofacial surgeons.

Maxillary sinus diseases

To be able to recognize sinus diseases, the dental surgeon should become familiar with the broad categories of sinus pathology. The maxillary sinus may be afflicted with a range of diseases, the most common of which are listed below.

INFECTIONS

1. Acute maxillary sinusitis.
2. Chronic maxillary sinusitis.

CYSTS

1. Antral lining cysts.
2. Odontogenic cysts.

BONE DYSPLASIAS

1. Fibrous dysplasia.
2. Paget's disease of bone.

BENIGN TUMOURS

1. Ossifying fibroma.
2. Osteoma (Gardner's syndrome).
3. Odontogenic tumours.

MALIGNANT TUMOURS

1. Squamous cell carcinoma.
2. Transitional cell carcinoma.
3. Osteosarcoma.
4. Invasive tumours:
      basal cell carcinoma
      salivary gland tumours.

Clinical presentation

Sinus pathology may sometimes mimic oral disease which may prompt the patient to visit a dentist first. The dental surgeon is then faced with the task of diagnosing a sinus problem or at least eliminating an oral cause. Disease of the maxillary sinus may present with one or more of the following clinical signs and symptoms.

- Facial pain – centred around the cheek and aggravated by coughing, exercise or bending forwards.
- Tenderness of the cheek to palpation, and of the posterior maxillary teeth to percussion.
- Swelling of the cheek, which is often erythematous. Occasionally there may be a palatal swelling.
- Nasal discharge, obstruction or epistaxis:
     infection – has a mucopurulent discharge
     tumour – may have a serosanguinous discharge.
- Oroantral communication – see above.
- Eye signs such as proptosis, diplopia or blocked nasolacrimal drainage resulting in epiphora.
- Altered sensation – over the cheek.

Investigations

To confirm a maxillary sinus disorder prior to referral, the dentist may wish to order sinus-related investigations, in particular certain plain X-ray views. Investigations that may be useful in the diagnosis of maxillary sinus pathology are as follows.

- **Intraoral radiographs** – where greater detail is required for sinus pathology of dental origin:
  - periapical dental X-ray
  - lateral or rotated maxillary occlusal.
- **Extraoral radiographs** – where the whole sinus cavity needs to be inspected for gross signs such as fluid levels, opacification, fractures and bony erosion of the sinus walls:
  - occipitomental 15 and 45 degrees
  - orthopantomogram
  - lateral skull or true lateral cephalogram
  - rotated lateral oblique 30 degrees.
- **Computerized tomography** (CT) – where a broader and clearer view of the sinus is required (particularly useful for complex midface fractures and suspected tumours):
  - axial views
  - coronal views
  - three-dimensional CT reconstructions.
- **Biopsy:**
  - aspiration – antral puncture best avoided in the presence of acute infection
  - endoscopy – fibreoptic technology allows direct visual inspection of sinus cavity and ability to procure tissue specimens with minimally invasive surgery.

Note: biopsy and CT scanning should be left to the specialist to arrange.

Recognizing maxillary sinus diseases

In addition to the clinical features mentioned previously, specific characteristic signs and symptoms of sinus disease may help the dental surgeon in arriving at a diagnosis. Since most of the sinus pathology also occurs in the oral cavity and jaws, only three specific maxillary sinus diseases are discussed in this chapter. The other related sinus diseases are discussed in more detail in Chapter 12.

MAXILLARY SINUSITIS

Causes

1. Upper respiratory tract infections.
2. Dental infections.
3. Oroantral communications.
4. Foreign body in sinus.
5. Interference with antral drainage, e.g. allergic rhinitis.
6. Facial trauma.

Pathogenesis
Bacterial or viral infection of the maxillary sinus results in inflammation of
the sinus lining.

Clinical features

- **Acute maxillary sinusitis:**
    throbbing pain, aggravated by head movements, stooping, coughing
    or sneezing
    toothache in maxillary molar/premolar region:
        all teeth respond vital
        tender to percussion
        premature tooth contact (teeth slightly extruded) causing tender-
        ness when chewing
    pyrexia and malaise
    mucopurulent nasal discharge and obstruction
    erythema and swelling of cheek
    fluid level apparent on plain radiographs (Figure 10.6).
- **Chronic maxillary sinusitis:**
    some tenderness of the cheek to palpation
    halitosis and postnasal drip
    obstruction of ostium which further aggravates problem
    mucosal hypertrophy of lining and polyp formation which shows up
    as opaque thickened sinus walls and cavity.

General management

- **Non-surgical:**
    bed rest

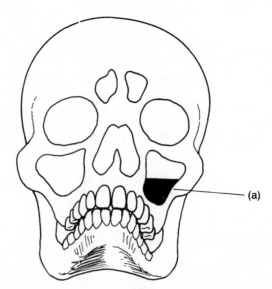

(a)

Figure 10.6 Diagram of Water's (occipitomental) view demonstrating fluid level in the left
maxillary sinus (a) indicative of acute sinusitis or blood in antrum secondary to midfacial
trauma.

adequate fluid intake
nasal decongestants (local and systemic)
mucolytic agents
antibiotics
analgesics.
- **Surgical:**
surgical drainage of pus and lavage of sinus cavity
intranasal antrostomy
radical antrectomy – Caldwell-Luc approach, reserved for intractable
cases.

ANTRAL LINING CYSTS

Antral lining cysts are found in 2–10% of routine orthopantomograms.
The aetiology is unknown.

Types
- **Secretory cysts:**
retention cysts of seromucous glands
prone to continuous enlargement
may erode bone by pressure atrophy.
- **Non-secretory cysts:**
arise from cystic degeneration of central areas of mucosal polyps
contain thin, yellowish fluid that drains into nose.

Pathology
The cysts arise in epithelial tissues of the sinus mucosa; they are only occasionally lined by epithelium.

Clinical features
Cysts are often asymptomatic and are usually found on routine radiography. Orthopantomograms show dome-shaped shadows in sinus 1–4 cm in
diameter (Figure 10.7).

Treatment
1. Radiographic follow-up is all that is usually required.
2. Aspiration is usually curative.
3. Surgically remove only if symptomatic or diagnosis is doubtful.

MALIGNANT TUMOURS OF THE MAXILLARY SINUS

The aetiology of malignant tumours is unknown.

Pathology
Eighty per cent of malignant tumours of the maxillary sinus are squamous
cell carcinomas arising from the sinus lining.

Clinical features
- **General features:**
often a late presentation

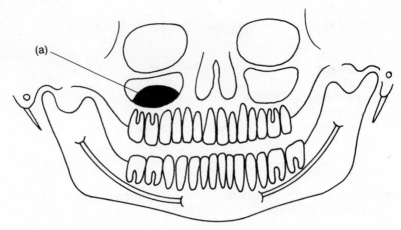

Figure 10.7 Diagram of orthopantomogram showing cyst (a) in right maxillary sinus as a low, domed, faintly radio-opaque but well-delineated structure.

    eye signs – proptosis, epiphora, diplopia
    nasal signs – obstruction, discharge, epistaxis
    cheek – swelling, ulceration of skin is a very late feature
    pain/paraesthesia – along distribution of maxillary nerve V_2.
- **Oral features** *(all dentists take careful note)*:
    swelling of alveolar ridge
    paraesthesia of buccal and palatal mucosa
    maxillary teeth:
        toothache
        non-vital
        displaced teeth creating a malocclusion
        abnormally mobile
        delayed healing of extraction sites – neoplastic tissue growing into
        extraction site.

Management and prognosis
Surgically resectable tumours have a 5-year survival rate of 45%. Unresectable tumours treated with radiotherapy have a 5-year survival rate of 12–19%. The overall 5-year survival rate is about 25%, compared with about 40% for oral cancer, since most maxillary sinus tumours present quite late.

Further reading

Howe GL (1985) *Minor Oral Surgery*. 3rd edn, pp 207–223. Oxford: Butterworth-Heinemann.
McGowan DA, Baxter PW, James J (1993) *The Maxillary Sinus and its Dental Implications*. Oxford: Butterworth-Heinemann.
Peterson LJ, Ellis III E, Hupp JR, Tucker MR (1993) *Contemporary Oral and Maxillofacial Surgery*. 2nd edn, pp 465–482. St Louis: Mosby.
Schow SR (1991) Infections of the maxillary sinus. In *Infections of the Head and Neck* (DM Laskin, RA Strauss, eds). *Oral Maxillofac Surg Clinics North Am*, **3**, 343–354.

11 Preprosthetic surgery

To facilitate the fabrication of a dental prosthesis, the edentulous alveolar base must be free of any disease or anatomical abnormalities that could compromise successful denture construction. In some instances, surgery may be necessary to alter an unfavourable anatomical or pathological feature. The aim of this chapter is to introduce the concept of preprosthetic surgery and to outline some examples of minor procedures that can be undertaken in an outpatient setting.

Terminology

Preprosthetic surgery – surgery that is undertaken to facilitate or aid in the construction of a successful dental prosthesis.

Aims of preprosthetic surgery

To secure a stable denture base in order to:

1. Simplify the design and construction of the dental prosthesis.
2. Enhance retention of a dental prosthesis.
3. Counteract displacing forces during a normal oral function.
4. Reduce the potential for adverse bone and soft tissue changes as a result of prosthetic function.

The ideal denture base

An important key to successful prosthetic rehabilitation lies in the construction of a prosthesis over an ideal edentulous base that boasts the following favourable features:

1. Broad convex ridge form.
2. Fixed tissues over residual alveolar ridge.
3. Adequate buccal and lingual sulcus depth.
4. Favourable inter-ridge relationships.
5. Adequate mandibular bone for strength and protection of the mandibular neurovascular bundle.
6. Arched palatal vault.
7. Post-tuberosity notch in maxilla to facilitate posterior border seal.

Classification of procedures

Minor preprosthetic surgery

The following conditions are often encountered in minor oral surgery practice and are discussed in further detail below.

- **Hard tissues:**
    alveolar bone abnormalities
    exostoses.
- **Soft tissues:**
    redundant and loose alveolar crestal tissue
    hyperplastic maxillary tuberosity
    mucosal fibrous hyperplasia
    palatal papillary hyperplasia
    prominent fraenum.

Major preprosthetic surgery

Discussion of major preprosthetic surgical procedures is beyond the scope of this book and so a further reading list is provided for those wishing to pursue this area in greater detail.

- **Relative augmentation of alveolar ridge:**
    vestibuloplasties.
- **Absolute augmentation of alveolar ridge:**
    bone grafts
    osteotomies.
- **Dental implants** (see Chapter 18):
    endosseous – osseointegrated screw implants
    transmandibular (Bosker) implants.

Alveolar bone abnormalities

Alveoloplasty refers to the surgical contouring of the alveolar ridge which may be undertaken as a primary procedure – i.e. at the time of the dental extractions – or may be done as a secondary procedure – i.e. after the alveolar ridge is fully healed following dental extractions. Alveoloplasty is the most commonly performed preprosthetic surgical procedure and is a technique that all clinicians should become familiar with.

Primary alveoloplasty

At the time of the dental extractions, the clinician must aim to preserve as much alveolar bone as possible and reduce the likelihood of unfavourable healing of the alveolar ridge by:

- Digital compression of the sockets after the teeth are removed to prevent the development of bony undercuts once the alveolus is healed.

- Avoiding surgical extractions as far as possible by cultivating an effective intra-alveolar forceps technique.
- Retaining both the buccal and lingual plates of bone and, wherever indicated, only removing the interseptal bone to promote rapid healing of the alveolus through primary closure (Figure 11.1).

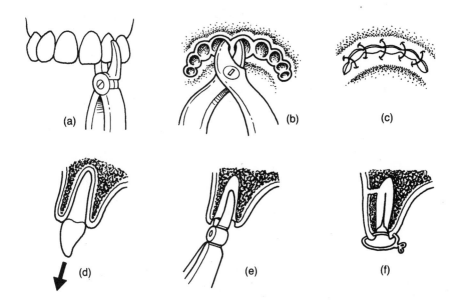

Figure 11.1 Primary alveoloplasty technique: a, careful extraction of teeth; b, removal of interseptal bone with bone rongeurs; c, compression of buccal alveolar plate with primary closure; d–f, steps a–c seen in cross-sectional view.

Secondary alveoloplasty

The alveolar ridge may require surgical recontouring some months or years following dental extractions in order to treat the following:

- Lateral bony projections or exostoses which create undercuts that prevent the denture from being seated properly. The bony projections may be surgically reduced with a bone file, chisel or burr through a crestal incision that is primarily closed at the end of the procedure (Figure 11.2).
- Sharp crestal bone can be smoothed over with a bone file, chisel or large round burr through a crestal incision.

Note: keep bone reduction to a minimum and always check the adequacy of the reduction by replacing the mucosa over the surgical site and feeling the resultant contour with your finger.

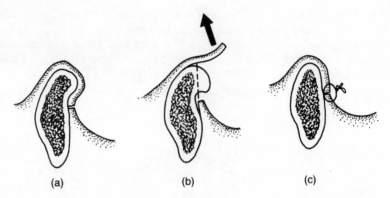

Figure 11.2 Secondary alveoloplasty: a, bony undercut on buccal aspect of mandibular alveolus; b, raising a buccal flap and removal of bony projection; c, primary closure.

Exostoses

Exostoses are common, non-neoplastic, localized overgrowths of normal lamellar bone which may result from trauma, chronic inflammation or often developmental anomaly such as a torus.

Torus palatinus

Torus palatinus occurs in about 20–25% of the population. It is a developmental anomaly of bone that presents as a discrete, rounded, painless bony swelling in the midline of the hard palate. It often interferes with the construction of an upper removable prosthesis that requires palatal coverage and so is frequently removed.

SURGICAL TECHNIQUE

The surgical removal of a palatal torus involves the following steps (Figure 11.3):

1. Construction of a surgical stent preoperatively with the torus reduced on the plaster model.
2. Lateral cephalogram X-ray investigation to see if torus is pneumatized, which may result in a large oronasal fistula if it is removed.
3. Exposure of torus via a sagittal incision with a forked 'Y' at each end to allow retraction of the mucosal flaps.
4. Reduction of bony torus – may be performed in a number of ways:
   using a large round burr – time-consuming
   using a chisel – may be imprecise and cause unwanted fractures to propagate beyond the actual torus
   scoring the torus in a cross-hatch pattern with a fissure burr then chiselling away one small section at a time
   combination of all three methods.

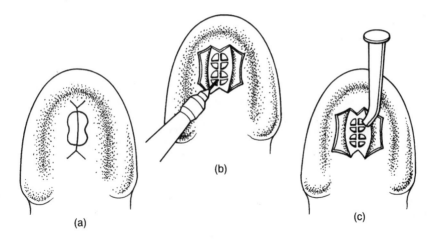

Figure 11.3 Surgical removal of palatal torus: a, double 'Y' incision over palatal torus; b, bony torus is first scored in a cross-hatch pattern with fissure burr; c, torus is removed with curved chisel and the base finally trimmed smooth with a large acrylic burr before the flaps are replaced.

5. Wound toilet and primary closure – the excess flap margins may have to be trimmed once the torus is removed.
6. Placement of a surgical stent for 3–5 days may be helpful in providing direct support to flaps and minimize the chance of a haematoma developing.

Torus mandibularis

Torus mandibularis is an evolutionary by-product of simian shelves which are commonly found in primates. Mandibular tori present as discrete, painless bony lumps on the lingual plate of the mandibular alveolus in the premolar region. They are found to occur bilaterally in 80% of cases. These often interfere with the lingual flange of a mandibular prosthesis and so removal is often recommended.

SURGICAL TECHNIQUE

The removal of a mandibular torus involves the following steps:

1. Alveolar crest incision along the premolar region and gentle exposure of the torus via a lingual flap which is often very delicate and liable to tearing.
2. Surgical reduction of the torus by:
    chisel – which is quick, and often can be performed accurately with minimal trauma to the lingual flap
    burr – more time-consuming and potentially more traumatic to the lingual flap.
3. Wound toilet and primary closure.

Alveolar crestal tissue

A patient who has been edentulous for many years may sometimes present with loose, ill-fitting dentures seated upon a loose and flabby alveolar ridge. This is often the case in patients with a maxillary denture opposing a natural mandibular dentition, which over many years has resulted in pressure resorption of alveolar bone in the anterior maxilla leaving behind redundant and mobile overlying mucosa. Provided there is no plan to augment the alveolar ridge, then surgical removal of the excess flabby tissue may be undertaken.

Surgical technique

Redundant and mobile crestal tissue is surgically removed as follows (Figure 11.4):

1. A narrow elliptical band of loose crestal tissue is removed by an elliptical incision into the mobile tissues on either side of the crest.
2. A submucous tissue wedge is excised under each side of the incision line.
3. The margins of the wound are directly apposed to create a new crest of alveolar mucosa and sutured together with horizontal mattress sutures.
4. As a temporary measure, the patient's existing denture may be lined with an interim denture relining material such as Viscogel until the tissues are sufficiently healed to commence construction of a new prosthesis.

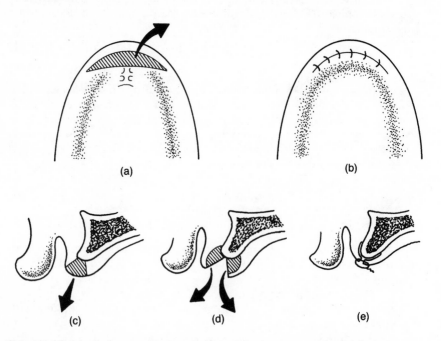

Figure 11.4 Removal of excess alveolar crest tissue: a, wedge-shaped excision of alveolar crest tissue; b, primary closure; c, cross-section – tissue wedge first removed; d, cross-section – resection of submucosal tissue; e, cross-section – primary closure.

Hyperplastic maxillary tuberosity

An enlarged maxillary tuberosity may interfere with the construction of a dental prosthesis by reducing the interocclusal space available to accommodate the artificial teeth. The hyperplasia may be due to overgrowth of dense fibrotic mucosal ridges, enlarged bony tuberosities, or combined bone and soft tissue overgrowth.

Surgical technique

The reduction of an enlarged maxillary tuberosity involves the following steps (Figure 11.5):

1. Preoperative X-rays are required to determine:
     the nature of the hyperplasia – bone, soft tissue or both
     if the bony tuberosity is pneumatized, which would increase the risk of oroantral communication with surgical reduction.
2. Soft tissue reduction:
     elliptical excision of crestal mucosa
     submucous wedge resection of underlying fibrotic tissue
     direct apposition of incision margins and closure with horizontal mattress sutures.

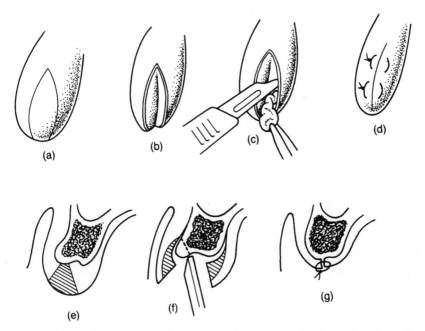

Figure 11.5 Reduction of hyperplastic maxillary tuberosity: a, wedge-shaped incision outline; b, tissue wedge removed; c, removal of submucosal tissue; d, primary closure with horizontal mattress sutures; e, cross-section – tissue wedge removed; f, cross-section – submucous resection and removal of bony undercuts; g, cross-section – primary closure.

3. Bony reduction:
    through a crestal incision the whole tuberosity is exposed
    the excess bone is reduced with a combination of bone file, chisel and
    burr
    primary closure with horizontal mattress sutures.

Mucosal fibrous hyperplasia (denture granuloma)

Broad-based, leaf-like folds of hyperplastic tissue surrounding the periphery
of an ill-fitting denture are often found in the labial mandibular sulcus
(Figure 11.6).

- **Aetiology** – possible causes include:
    ill-fitting dentures
    dentures with over-extended labial flanges
    chronic resorption of alveolar ridge without concomitant adjustments
    to original denture, i.e. no trimming of the flanges as the denture
    settles with changes in alveolar height over many years.

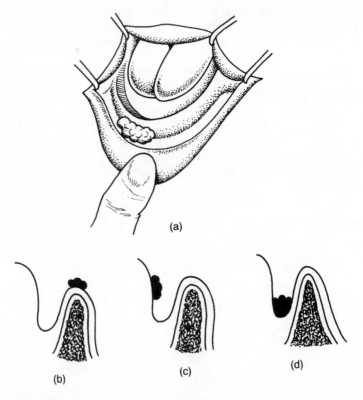

Figure 11.6 Mucosal fibrous hyperplasia: a, hyperplastic tissue in mandibular labial sulcus;
b, type 1 – hyperplastic tissue on alveolar ridge; c, type 2 – hyperplastic tissue outside
denture-bearing area; d, type 3 – hyperplastic tissue at the base of the sulcus (most difficult
to remove since there is a great risk of losing essential sulcus depth postoperatively).

- **Pathogenesis** – repeated trauma and ulceration of labial mucosa resulting from chronic irritation from the denture periphery leads to exuberant formation of granulation tissue which heals with hyperplastic scarring.

Presurgical preparation

1. Denture adjustment – trim back the overextended flanges so that denture is not in direct contact with hyperplastic tissue.
2. Prescribe a regimen of chlorhexidine and salt-water mouth rinses for at least 2–3 weeks before planned surgery.
3. The above measures serve to eliminate any signs of inflammation and in many cases result in marked reduction of the hyperplastic tissue; this facilitates less drastic surgery and favours better healing postoperatively.

Surgical technique

Hyperplastic tissue is eliminated by:

1. Sharp dissection of hyperplastic tissues – which should always be submitted for histopathological examination.
2. Primary closure of the resultant wound if the excision is small. For more extensive excisions it may be necessary to close the wound with:
   local flaps
   free mucosal or skin grafts which may be held in place by soft tissue trimmed dentures wired to the jaws.
3. Cryosurgery and laser surgery have been used with much success and are purported to result in reduced postoperative pain and little scar formation.

Note: healing by secondary intention must be avoided as this will adversely reduce the sulcus depth and hence compromise denture stability.

Palatal papillary hyperplasia

In palatal papillary hyperplasia numerous small, tightly packed papillary projections are seen, over part or all of the denture-bearing area of the palate. The palate has an inflamed, 'pebbled' appearance.

- **Aetiology** – unknown; may be related to a combination of:
   ill-fitting dentures
   poor denture hygiene and continuous wearing
   chronic candidal infection.

Presurgical preparation

1. Advice on denture hygiene (overnight chlorhexidine denture soak) and leaving dentures out of mouth as much as possible.
2. Antifungal chemotherapy – amphotericin lozenges 10 mg dissolved in mouth four times daily for up to 3–4 weeks.

3. Salt-water and chlorhexidine mouth washes.
4. Recommendation for construction of new dentures after surgery.

Surgical technique

Once all signs of inflammation are eliminated, the papillary hyperplasia may be treated in one of a number of ways.

SHARP DISSECTION

A sharp antral curette is used. Protect the resultant surgical wound with a soft tissue liner and allow 3–5 weeks for healing by secondary epithelialization.

MUCOABRASION

Mucoabrasion is performed using an acrylic burr or a rotating wire brush, with the same postoperative regimen as above. This technique often results in poor surface morphology of the palatal vault.

ELECTROCAUTERY

The full-thickness burn resulting from electrocautery may be painful postoperatively, and necrotic tissues are easily infected if meticulous oral hygiene is not maintained.

CRYOSURGERY

Cryosurgery can easily be done on an outpatient basis. There is relatively little postoperative pain as the hyperplastic tissue necroses and peels off in a few weeks to create a smooth palatal surface.

LASER SURGERY

Tissues can be more accurately sculptured with minimal postoperative pain, oedema, bleeding and scarring. Patient must keep extremely still when laser is active to avoid inadvertent movement of the beam causing damage to adjacent tissues. The requirement for high technology and expensive equipment may limit its more widespread use.

Prominent fraenum

Occasionally, the labial, buccal or lingual fraena may interfere with denture construction, particularly where they attach close to the crest of the alveolus. A point of weakness is thus introduced to the denture in places where it has been excessively relieved or trimmed back to accommodate a prominent fraenum. If not adequately relieved, the denture will be displaced during function by the action of the fraena. In these situations the fraena are best reduced or completely removed.

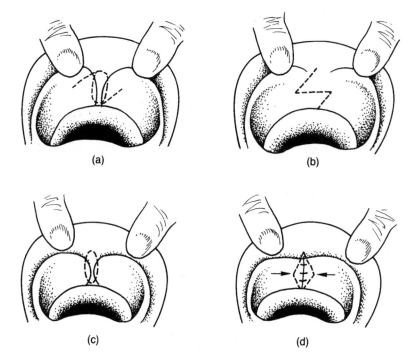

Figure 11.7 Surgical management of fraenum: a, fraenoplasty – incision outline; b, Z-plasty closure; c, fraenectomy outline; d, undermining of tissues and direct primary closure.

Surgical technique

There are two ways of treating prominent fraena (Figure 11.7).

FRAENOPLASTY

Plastic surgical procedures are used to alter the size and shape of the fraenum so that it becomes less prominent.

- **Z-plasty** – reorients the direction of the tension band.
- **V–Y advancement** – places the fraena attachment apically away from the crest of the ridge.

FRAENECTOMY

Fraenectomy is the complete removal of the fraenum through a diamond-shaped excision and primary closure of the margins.

Ankyloglossia

Where there is a prominent lingual fraenum resulting in tongue tie and significant denture relief to avoid displacement of the denture during function, then a lingual fraenectomy is recommended. This is achieved by releasing the fraenum close to the tongue, which will prevent accidental cutting of the submandibular duct and orifice.

Conclusion

When contemplating the need for preprosthetic surgery, the clinician must balance the benefits of surgery against the morbidity and inconvenience it creates for the patient. Many of the patients likely to be considered for pre-prosthetic surgery are elderly and frail, and even relatively minor surgery can be a serious undertaking for these patients. In many instances an experienced clinician can construct an adequate denture that will obviate the need for surgery, even in the presence of some unfavourable anatomical or pathological conditions.

Further reading

Fonseca RJ, Davis WH (1995) *Reconstructive Preprosthetic Oral and Maxillofacial Surgery.* 2nd edn. Philadelphia: Saunders.

Hopkins R (1990) *A Colour Atlas of Preprosthetic Oral Surgery.* London: Wolfe.

Koerner KR, Tilt LV, Johnson KR (1994) *Color Atlas of Minor Oral Surgery.* London: Mosby-Wolfe.

Peterson LJ, Ellis III E, Hupp JR, Tucker MR (1993) *Contemporary Oral and Maxillofacial Surgery.* 2nd edn, pp 295–330. St Louis: Mosby.

12 Surgical oral pathology

Surgery has a dual role in relation to oral pathology and oral medicine. Firstly, surgery is used as a means of procuring tissues for histopathological examination and diagnosis. Secondly, and more importantly, surgery is used as a means of treating pathological conditions by physically removing the diseased tissues, thereby achieving a cure. A thorough understanding of pathology is an essential attribute of a successful surgeon.

Oral pathology and oral medicine are extensive subjects in their own right. It is beyond the scope of this book to pursue any detailed discussion of oral diseases. Instead, the reader is encouraged to consult the reading list provided at the end of this chapter. In this chapter the discussion focuses on the role of minor oral surgery in relation to oral disease.

Much of what is described has more relevance to the senior house officer in oral and maxillofacial surgery than to the general dentist. However, all dentists must be cognisant with the clinical presentation of the more common oral diseases since prompt referral for specialist management is essential. Treatment procedures described are purely for general information and should never be attempted without proper clinical supervision and adequate hospital training.

Terminology

Oral pathology – a branch of dentistry that deals with the study and diagnosis of oral disease, i.e. diseases of the mouth, jaws and associated structures. There is a trend to rename the discipline 'oral and maxillofacial pathology'.
Oral medicine – a branch of dentistry that deals with the diagnosis and non-surgical management of diseases of the oral cavity and associated structures (excluding the teeth).
Biopsy – a tissue specimen that is surgically removed for the purposes of histopathological examination.
Surgical pathology – diseases that are amenable to surgical treatment.

Classification of human diseases

All human disease may be classified into one of the following broad categories:

- **Congenital** – a disorder, usually a morphological tissue defect, that is present at the time of birth (e.g. cleft lip and palate):
    isolated
    part of a syndrome.
- **Developmental** – a disorder that arises some months or years after birth (e.g. dentigerous cyst):
    genetic (e.g. metabolic and endocrine disorders)
    acquired (e.g. degenerative disorders).
- **Traumatic** – a disorder that results from a noxious physical event that disrupts normal tissue architecture, growth and development (e.g. dilacerated incisor):
    accidental
    surgical.
- **Inflammatory** – a disease arising from a tissue reaction to an endogenous or exogenous stimulus (e.g. oral lichen planus):
    infection
    autoimmune disorder
    hypersensitivity.
- **Neoplastic** – a disease arising from an abnormal mass of cells that fail to respond, for whatever reason, to normal environmental stimuli that control their growth, movement and differentiation (e.g. oral cancer):
    benign
    premalignant
    malignant.

Surgical objectives

When dealing with surgical pathology the fundamental objectives of surgery are as follows:

1. To eradicate the entire pathological lesion.
2. To leave no pathological tissues that could develop and lead to a recurrence.
3. To minimize collateral damage of normal surrounding tissues as a result of the surgery.
4. To promote rapid healing and restoration of function.

Factors that influence surgical planning

When surgeons decide on the best surgical approach to the management of a pathological lesion, the following factors are often considered:

1. The age and life expectancy of the patient.
2. General health of the patient – i.e. ability to tolerate the surgery.
3. Aggressiveness of the lesion – i.e. the destructive potential of the lesion. With malignant disease, the best and often the only chance of cure is with the first operation.
4. Size and location of the lesion – proximity of the lesion to vital structures such as nerves and major blood vessels or organs.

5. Anticipated recurrence potential of the lesion – cure or palliation.
6. The surgical defect produced – can function and aesthetic appearance be acceptably restored?

Managing pathology in minor oral surgery practice

When a dental surgeon encounters minor pathological conditions within the oral cavity or jaws, the surgical objectives and treatment planning principles remain the same as those of the specialist surgeon treating major disease. Only dental surgeons with adequate hospital experience and clinical training (at least to the level of senior house officer in oral and maxillofacial surgery) may usefully participate in the care of patients presenting with oral pathology, in the following ways.

Diagnosis

- Ordering further investigations – blood tests, radiographs, etc. (see Chapters 2 and 17).
- Providing tissue specimens for the pathologist, such as:
    aspirate
        fine needle for solid lesions
        wide-bore needle for cystic lesions
    cytology
        scraping
        smear
    tissue biopsy
        incisional
        excisional
        drill biopsy.

Note: in general dental practice fine needle aspiration, excisional and drill biopsies are best referred to the experts.

Treatment

In the best interests of patient care a pathological lesion should only be treated by experienced senior house officers in the following circumstances:

1. Lesion is less than 1 cm across and is not malignant.
2. Lesion is easily accessible – i.e. in the anterior part of the mouth.
3. There are no important anatomical structures in close proximity with the lesion, e.g. inferior dental canal, mental foramen, sinus cavity.
4. The procedure can be performed under local anaesthesia.
5. The clinician has previously undertaken the surgery under specialist supervision.
6. The well-informed, consenting patient fully understands the limited surgical expertise of the treating clinician.

Aiding the pathologist

Using tissue specimens provided by the surgeon, the pathologist is able to determine the nature, pathology and diagnosis of the lesion at the light microscopic level. However, an accurate histopathological diagnosis is often difficult to achieve without an adequate tissue specimen and a complete clinical history and description of the lesion. The surgeon should therefore provide the pathologist with the following details (Figure 12.1):

ORAL PATHOLOGY DIAGNOSTIC SERVICE
HISTOPATHOLOGY / CYTOLOGY REQUEST FORM

PATIENT DETAILS:

Surname_____*JONES*_____

Given Names_____*PETER*_____

Date of Birth *20 / 12 / 74*____ Age *20*____ Sex *Male*

Home Address ___*123 Somewhere St ANYWHERE 54321*

Daytime Contact Telephone____*654 3210*____

CLINICIAN DETAILS:

Name_____*JOHN SMITH*____*Oral + Maxillofacial Surgeon*

Practice Address_____

Telephone No._____ Fax No._____

HISTORY OF LESION   *Palatal Swelling   1 week duration*
                    Left side - Anterior

BIOPSY SITE *Left Premaxilla via palatal flap*

DESCRIPTION OF LESION
(include sketch where possible)   *left palatal Swelling*

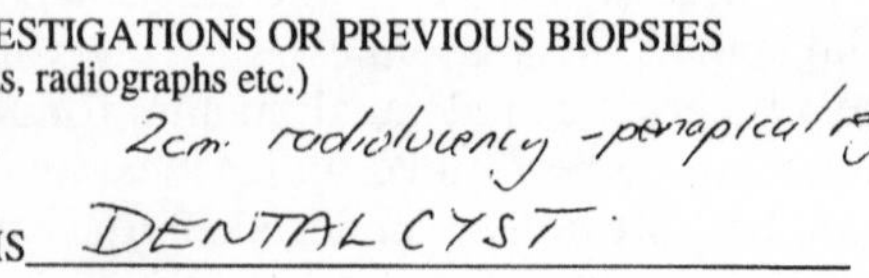

TYPE OF SPECIMEN - Tick appropriate box.
          Incisional biopsy []   Excisional biopsy [✓]   Smear []   Aspirate []

RESULTS OF OTHER INVESTIGATIONS OR PREVIOUS BIOPSIES
     (ie: dental vitality tests, radiographs etc.)
          Non vital /2   2cm. radiolucency -periapical region of /2

PROVISIONAL DIAGNOSIS___*DENTAL CYST*_____

Date of Biopsy ___*1 / 10 / 1995*___.

Figure 12.1 Pathology request form.

1. Patient details – age and sex. Brief medical history such as current medication and chronic illnesses may be sometimes useful.
2. Historical summary – possible cause (e.g. trauma), duration, changes in size, shape or colour.
3. Clinical symptoms – pain, altered sensation, limited mouth opening, difficulty chewing or talking, limited tongue movements, halitosis.
4. Clinical signs – location, size, shape, consistency, surface, discharge. A simple drawing of the lesion will aid immensely in its description.
5. Results of other investigations – blood tests, radiographs.
6. Adequate biopsy specimen:
    enough tissue procured to allow adequate representation of the disease
    delicate handling of tissue biopsy specimen to minimize trauma
    tissue kept moist or placed immediately into suitable fixative such as 10% formol saline.
7. Date (and occasionally time) of biopsy.
8. Orientation of the biopsy specimen in relation to adjacent tissues. Common practice is to mark one side of the specimen with a silk suture so that biopsy may be oriented in relation to the position of the suture.

Note: it is prudent to enlist the services of a pathology laboratory that has an oral pathologist on the staff, since a general pathologist who has little interest or experience in oral pathology may provide a report with conflicting terminology. The worst scenario is the diagnosis of malignancy in a benign lesion such as chronic sialometaplasia.

Oral diseases

Diseases that afflict the human body in general may also be found in the oral cavity, jaws and associated tissues. To illustrate the role of minor oral surgery in the management of oral pathology, examples of some common oral diseases are used, under the following headings:

1. Cysts.
2. Pathology of the oral mucosa.
3. Pathology of the jaws.
4. Pathology of the salivary glands.

Cysts

A cyst is a pathological cavity which is not created by the accumulation of pus and contains fluid, semifluid or gaseous substances (after Kramer 1974).

CLASSIFICATION OF ORAL CYSTS

Soft tissue cysts

• Salivary mucocele, e.g. mucus retention or extravasation cysts.
• Skin, e.g. epidermoid or dermoid cysts.

- Lymphoepithelial cysts.
- Thyroglossal cysts.

Cysts of the jaws

- **Epithelial lined cysts:**
    developmental
        odontogenic, e.g. keratocyst, dentigerous cyst
        non-odontogenic, e.g. nasopalatine (incisive canal) duct cyst
    inflammatory, e.g. dental cyst.
- **Non-epithelial cysts:**
    simple bone cyst (traumatic, solitary, haemorrhagic)
    aneurysmal bone cyst.

CLINICAL PRESENTATION OF ORAL CYSTS

1. Discrete swelling in oral cavity.
2. Displacement of teeth and altered occlusion – e.g. keratocyst.
3. Missing teeth – e.g. dentigerous cyst.
4. Loose teeth.
5. Non-vital teeth – e.g. dental cyst.
6. Ill-fitting dentures – e.g. residual cyst.
7. Pain and tenderness – only when cyst is infected.
8. Pathological fractures – particularly with large jaw cysts.
9. Facial asymmetry – large jaw cysts.
10. Mental nerve paraesthesia – rare, but may arise from pressure effects of large cyst.

NON-SURGICAL INVESTIGATIONS

When confronted with a clinical presentation suggestive of an oral cyst, the following non-surgical investigations may be performed to aid in the diagnosis.

Plain X-rays
Plain X-ray films are useful for cysts of the jaws.

- Orthopantomogram – an excellent general screening film that will show the full size of the cyst as well as cysts in multiple sites.
- Dental radiographs – good for demonstrating the detailed relationship of a cyst with a nearby tooth or teeth.

Vitality testing
Vitality testing of teeth is important in confirming the diagnosis of a dental cyst, especially with lesions closely associated with teeth.

Computerized axial tomography
Computerized tomographic scanning is reserved for extremely large and destructive jaw cysts that extend beyond the confines of the jaws and spill out into soft tissues. *Refer to hospital.*

Ultrasonography
Ultrasound scanning is helpful in determining the cystic nature of large soft tissue lesions such as a plunging ranula. *Refer to hospital.*

IMPORTANT RADIOLOGICAL FEATURES OF JAW CYSTS

When examining radiographs of cystic lesions, it is prudent to observe and note the following important features:

1. Size, shape, number and the sites of the radiolucencies.
2. Margins of the radiolucency – well-delineated, sclerotic, ill-defined or merging with surrounding bone.
3. Teeth – look for displacement or resorption of the roots.
4. Areas of radio-opacity within the lumen of the 'cystic' lesion.
5. Displacement of the inferior alveolar neurovascular bundle.

SURGICAL INVESTIGATIONS

For a more definitive diagnosis, surgery may be used to obtain tissue specimens as follows.

Aspiration
Aspiration is a simple procedure that is used to determine the consistency within a 'cystic' lesion, i.e. solid, fluid or gaseous, which may occasionally be diagnostic in cases such as keratocysts (low protein content, $<4\,g/100\,ml$) and simple bone cysts (air or serosanguineous fluid). The importance of aspiration prior to definitive surgery is evident when in some cases the 'cystic' lesion may in fact be a vascular anomaly that will require a very different approach.

- **Technique:**
     under local anaesthetic a wide-bore needle (18 gauge) attached to a syringe is inserted into the lesion
     a second needle is inserted to act as an air inlet to allow aspiration of cyst contents
     risk of infection may render subsequent histopathology difficult to interpret, so aspiration is best done within 48 hours of definitive surgery with prophylactic antibiotics.

Biopsy
Biopsy is particularly important when large lesions are present (incisional biopsy). With small lesions, it is best to remove the whole cyst (excisional biopsy) for patient comfort and convenience and send the whole specimen for examination.

- **Technique for incisional biopsy:**
     use local anaesthesia
     soft tissue cysts – incise the overlying mucosa and expose the cyst wall through blunt dissection. Excise a small tissue specimen from the cyst lining

jaw cysts – raise a small flap. Make a window in the bone and gently remove the buccal plate of bone to expose the cyst lining. Excise a piece of cyst lining for biopsy

note that in many cases the biopsy procedure may form part of the definitive management of a cyst by utilizing the technique of decompression and marsupialization, discussed below.

PRINCIPLES OF SURGICAL MANAGEMENT

Cysts of the oral cavity and jaws can be managed in a number of ways. This is best left to specialist surgeons or hospital oral and maxillofacial surgery departments.

Enucleation
Enucleation is the complete shelling out of a cyst wall and its contents by:

curettage – piecemeal removal of a cyst wall and its contents from its bony or soft tissue surroundings by blunt dissection and scooping action of curettes, or

excision – cutting out a cyst wall and its contents together with its bony or soft tissue surroundings.

- **Advantages:**
  all pathological tissue is removed
  little patient compliance required postoperatively.
- **Disadvantages:**
  technically a very difficult procedure
  greater morbidity to surrounding structures.
- **Contraindications:**
  large cysts close to delicate structures such as vital tooth roots, interdental nerve
  existing pathological fracture.
- **Enucleation with primary closure:**
  the margins of the flap should rest on sound bone.
- **Enucleation with open packing:**
  instead of primary closure of the flap, or where there is no bone to support the line of incision, the flap is turned into the bone cavity with a 1.25 cm antiseptic-soaked gauze pack fixed in situ for 10 days.

Marsupialization
Marsupialization is the creation of a permanent opening from the cyst cavity into the mouth (Figure 12.2).

- **Indications:**
  for very large cysts where enucleation may cause unacceptable morbidity of surrounding vital structures, i.e. vital teeth.
- **Advantages:**
  technically much simpler than enucleation.
- **Disadvantages:**
  pathological tissue left in situ

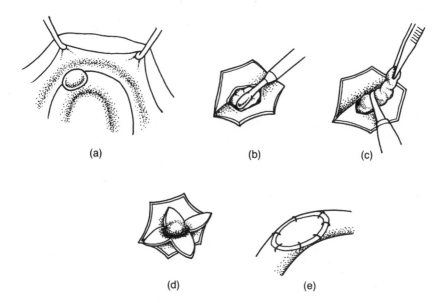

Figure 12.2 Surgical management of jaw cysts: a, cyst arising from edentulous maxillary alveolus; b, flap raised and bony covering carefully removed; c, cyst lining is gently separated from bony cavity with a fine periosteal elevator or curette; d, marsupialization of large cyst with incision and display of internal cyst lining; e, excess cyst lining trimmed and sutured to the surrounding oral mucosa to create a pouch (i.e. marsupialization).

requires considerable patient cooperation in keeping the cavity clean and the opening patent.

- **Technique:**

  a mucosal flap is raised. Blunt dissection of the mucosa from the cyst wall may be needed

  an H-shaped incision is made across the exposed cyst wall so that the cyst lining can be turned over and sutured to the periphery

  incision biopsy is taken of cyst wall

  cavity is packed with ribbon gauze soaked in antiseptic which is changed 10 days later

  packs should be changed at weekly intervals

  a removable acrylic obturator may be constructed which can be removed by the patient for regular cleaning. It must be adjusted regularly as the cavity shrinks in size.

Decompression

Decompression is a variant of marsupialization (see above).

- **Technique:**

  the operative procedure is limited to the removal of a small part of the cyst wall which is sent off as a biopsy specimen

  the small opening is kept patent until bone regeneration occurs and the cavity reduces in size; enucleation can then be undertaken on a much smaller lesion with less morbidity.

CYSTS IN MINOR ORAL SURGERY PRACTICE

On occasions the dental surgeon may be called upon to diagnose cystic lesions of the mouth and jaws when these appear during routine examination and on X-rays (Figure 12.3).

Diagnosis
Occasionally the dental surgeon may come across oral cysts, either in symptomatic patients or by chance finding on radiographs in asymptomatic patients. In either case the dental surgeon must follow the logical sequence of history, examination and investigations to arrive at a provisional diagnosis as outlined previously. The next step is to inform the patient and then refer the individual for specialist management.

Management
The oral and maxillofacial surgeon may elect to undertake the surgical management of the following lesions.

● **Dental cysts:**
   treated by enucleation and extraction or pulp extirpation and root canal obliteration of offending tooth
   see 'apicectomies' in Chapter 9.

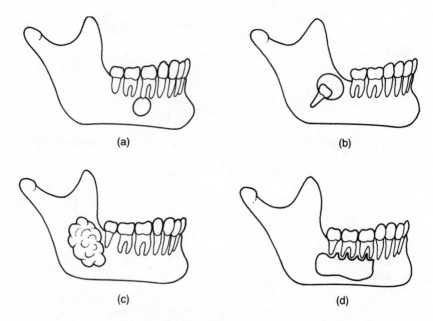

(a)   (b)

(c)   (d)

Figure 12.3 Radiographic features of radiolucent lesions of the mandible: a, periapical radiolucency – dental cyst; b, pericoronal radiolucency – dentigerous cyst; c, multiloculated radiolucency – keratocyst; d, scalloped radiolucency – simple bone cyst.

- **Dentigerous cysts:**
  removed at the same time as the associated impacted tooth is surgically removed
  tooth may be retained and cyst surgically excised if performed during active eruption phase of what may become a useful and functional tooth.
- **Paradental cysts:**
  enucleated together with the impacted wisdom tooth.
- **Residual cysts:**
  alveolar crestal incision with a buccal relieving incision
  removal of bone overlying cyst
  enucleation
  recurrence is rare.
- **Gingival cysts:**
  enucleation.
- **Lateral periodontal cysts:**
  enucleation.
- **Nasopalatine cyst:**
  palatal flap raised with sacrifice of nasopalatine nerves
  enucleation
  wound dehiscence is common – the site must be kept clean.

Pathology of the oral mucosa

Pathological conditions arising from the oral mucosa may be classified as surgical or non-surgical.

SURGICAL PATHOLOGY

Biopsies of the lesion may be performed in the following ways (Figure 12.4).

Excisional biopsy

Excisional biopsy is performed when the lesion is small enough to be totally removed, and the surgical defect can be easily repaired with primary closure. In this way, the whole specimen is available for histopathological examination.

A successful excisional biopsy must also contain a rim or border of normal tissue to indicate that no pathological tissue has been left behind.

Incisional biopsy

1. Where the lesion is larger than 1 cm or the resulting defect cannot be closed primarily, only a small representative portion of the lesion is excised as a biopsy.
2. In most cases, it is best to biopsy the edge of the lesion so that the specimen can include a portion of normal tissue to help the pathologist with the diagnosis.
3. The depth of the biopsy must include the epithelial basement membrane and part of the lamina propria of the underlying connective tissue.

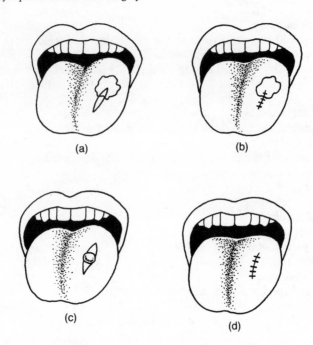

Figure 12.4 Biopsy techniques of tongue lesions: a, incisional biopsy – elliptical incision at the edge of the lesion incorporating a section of normal surrounding tissue; b, primary closure after incisional biopsy; c, excisional biopsy of small pedunculated mass; d, primary closure after complete removal of lesion.

4. Some surgeons use vital staining agents such as gentian violet to show up areas of dysplasia being considered for biopsy. Unfortunately, the staining highlights areas of inflammation in addition to dysplasia, therefore limiting the usefulness of this technique.

Punch biopsy

Punch biopsy is another form of incisional biopsy:

a sharp pair of tissue forceps is used in a grasping and rotating motion to extricate a small piece of tissue for biopsy
useful for multiple biopsies of suspected malignant lesions in poorly accessible areas such as the oropharynx.

NON-SURGICAL PATHOLOGY

Lesions that cannot be treated by surgery fall into the realm of oral medicine. The type of pharmacotherapy used to treat the lesions depends on the underlying disease, which is diagnosed with the aid of tissue specimens procured in the following ways.

Aspiration

Using a fine-gauge needle it may be possible to obtain vesicular fluid from the lesions in certain vesiculobullous disorders, which is then examined for characteristic cells or the presence of viruses.

Scraping

Using a sterile wooden spatula, scrape the surface of the lesion in one direction several times to obtain specimens of cells for cytological examination.

Often an adjunctive biopsy is also necessary to confirm the diagnosis, since this technique does not provide enough tissue evidence for definitive diagnosis.

This method is particularly useful for suspected candidal infections. The specimen obtained is spread across a microscopic glass slide, dried, fixed and then stained to check for the presence of hyphae.

Incisional biopsy

Incisional biopsy provides the definitive diagnosis.

The technique is the same as for surgical pathology, but check to see if immunofluorescent studies are required (e.g. for oral lichen planus) in which case a fresh biopsy specimen must be provided for the pathologist.

When tackling vesiculobullous lesions, try to ensure the biopsy specimen includes an intact vesicle or bulla, and always include a margin of normal tissue.

Pathology of the jaws

The management of jaw cysts has already been discussed (see above).

CLASSIFICATION OF JAW DISEASE

Jaw pathology may be broadly subdivided into the following disease categories.

Fibro-osseous lesions of the jaws

Whenever a biopsy is obtained from a suspected fibro-osseous lesion of the jaws, it is essential to provide the pathologist with the following details, which will permit a more accurate diagnosis to be made:

1. Clinical details.
2. Radiographs.
3. Serum chemistry:
        serum calcium and phosphate levels
        serum alkaline phosphatase level.

Odontogenic tumours

Odontogenic tumours are rare lesions which arise from the odontogenic apparatus. Many of these lesions are not true neoplasms but developmental anomalies composed of tissues derived from the tooth germ.

Primary bone tumours

Ranging from the benign osteoma to the rapidly destructive and malignant osteosarcoma, primary bone tumours are rare, although vigilant screening of patients may yield a chance finding every once in a while.

Haematopoietic tumours

Haematopoietic tumours are tumours in bone that arise from neoplastic cells normally found in the blood and bone marrow such as plasma cells (i.e. multiple myeloma) and eosinophils (solitary eosinophilic granuloma).

CLINICAL PRESENTATION

Jaw disease may present with one or more of the following clinical features:

1. Firm swelling of the buccal plate or palate.
2. Facial asymmetry.
3. Displaced teeth with malocclusion.
4. Loose or non-vital teeth.
5. Mental or infraorbital nerve paraesthesia.
6. Pathological fracture – especially lytic or destructive lesions.

RADIOGRAPHIC PRESENTATION

Jaw disorders are often asymptomatic and commonly picked up on routine radiographs. The radiographic appearance may vary.

- **Radiolucent lesion:**
  well circumscribed – well-defined sclerotic boundaries (central giant cell lesion)
  poorly circumscribed – ill-defined 'fuzzy' edges (ossifying/cementifying fibroma)
  multilocular (ameloblastoma)
  irregular outline (simple bone cyst)
  central radio-opacity (ameloblastic fibro-odontoma)
  'soap bubble' (odontogenic myxoma)
  punched-out (multiple myeloma).
- **Radio-opaque lesion:**
  well circumscribed (odontoma)
  'ground glass' appearance (fibrous dysplasia)
  'sunray' effect (osteosarcoma).
- **Dental features:**
  root resorption (ameloblastoma)
  widened periodontal ligament (osteosarcoma)
  sclerotic periapical lesion (cementoblastoma).
- **Inferior dental canal:**
  displaced
  widened canal.

BIOPSY OF JAW LESIONS

A mucoperiosteal flap is raised and a pathology specimen obtained by:

- Drill biopsy – a special biopsy drill is mounted on a surgical handpiece and used to obtain core type specimens.
- Curetting – particularly where the bone lesions are soft, such as the haematopoietic tumours.

TREATMENT OF JAW LESIONS

Jaw lesions can be surgically treated in the following ways (Figure 12.5).

Curettage
Curettage is the piecemeal removal of a soft lesion from its bony surroundings. It is reserved for lesions that do not recur even if not completely
removed, e.g. adenomatoid odontogenic tumour (AOT).

Enucleation
Enucleation is the complete shelling out of a lesion in one piece from its
bony surroundings, e.g. a complex odontoma.

Excision
Excision involves the removal of a lesion together with the bony walls
immediately surrounding the lesion, e.g. an osteoma.

Resection
Resection is the complete removal of the lesion together with varying
amounts of normal adjacent bone (partial, marginal or total) and
surrounding soft tissues (composite resection) – e.g. ameloblastoma or
osteosarcoma.

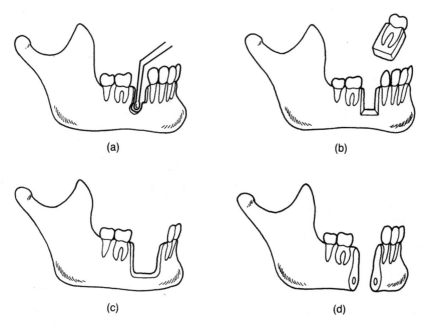

(a)

(b)

(c)

(d)

Figure 12.5 Surgical techniques used for the management of jaw lesions: a, curettage,
enucleation; b, excision; c, marginal resection; d, partial resection.

JAW PATHOLOGY AND MINOR ORAL SURGERY

Minor oral surgery for jaw disease is mainly confined to small biopsies and the curettage or enucleation of small benign and accessible bony lesions less than 1 cm in diameter.

Pathology of the salivary glands

Both major and minor salivary glands may be afflicted with disorders that occasionally may be picked up by the dental surgeon.

CLASSIFICATION OF SALIVARY GLAND DISORDERS

The spectrum of disorders that occur in the salivary glands may be classified under the following broad categories.

Congenital

1. Aplasia.
2. Hypoplasia (often part of a syndrome such as Treacher–Collins).

Inflammatory (sialadenitis)

1. Infection – bacterial, viral.
2. Autoimmune – Sjögren's syndrome.
3. Idiopathic – necrotizing sialometaplasia, sarcoidosis.

Traumatic

1. Mucocele or ranula.
2. Salivary fistula.
3. Postirradiation sialadenitis.

Obstructive

1. Sialolithiasis.
2. Atresia or ductal stenosis.

Salivary gland tumours

1. Benign, e.g. pleomorphic adenoma.
2. Malignant, e.g. adenoid cystic carcinoma.

Idiopathic

1. Sialosis.

CLINICAL PRESENTATION OF SALIVARY GLAND DISEASE

Swelling is the most common feature of salivary gland disease.

- **Common sites of swellings:**
  lower lip, e.g. mucocele
  upper lip, e.g. benign tumours (monomorphic adenomas)

junction of hard and soft palate, e.g. tumours or necrotizing sialometaplasia
floor of mouth, e.g. lesions of the sublingual gland such as a ranula
submandibular triangle, e.g. lesions of the submandibular gland
angle of mandible, e.g. parotid lesions.

- **History of swellings:**
  acute swellings – most likely to be acute sialadenitis associated with
  bacterial or viral infections
  recurrent swellings – most likely to be due to:
    trauma (e.g. mucocele, salivary fistula)
    obstruction of the salivary duct or papilla (e.g. calculus, atresia,
    fibrosis)
    gland distension (e.g. allergy or adverse drug reaction such as
    iodine sensitivity)
  persistent swellings:
    diffuse – may be due to Sjögren's syndrome, sialosis or sarcoidosis
    nodular enlargement – most likely to be a neoplastic lesion, benign
    if slow-growing over many years, or malignant if rapid growth
    over a few months.

SALIVARY GLAND INVESTIGATIONS

Diagnosis of salivary gland disorders may be further aided by the following
investigations which are best left to the experts.

- **Plain X-rays:**
  most commonly used for detection of salivary calculi
  examples include lower occlusal view, orthopantomograph, lateral
  oblique view of the mandible for submandibular calculi, and anteroposterior mandibular views for parotid stones.
- **Sialography:**
  the internal duct system of the gland is delineated through the use of
  radio-opaque contrast solution injected into the gland
  employed where there are duct strictures or dilatations, small or
  radiolucent stones and salivary fistulae.
- **CT scans:**
  sometimes combined with sialography techniques
  because of expense, complexity and radiation, best reserved for
  suspected neoplastic lesions of the salivary glands.
- **Magnetic resonance imaging (MRI):**
  limited availability and high cost have restricted the use of this investigation to large hospitals and teaching institutions
  lack of ionizing radiation and good soft tissue detail makes this a
  promising adjunctive and eventually an alternative to CT scans for
  neoplastic disorders of the salivary glands.
- **Radionucleotide salivary scanning:**
  part of nuclear medicine
  provides valuable information on the functional and (to a lesser
  extent) the anatomical status of the diseased major glands. Unfortunately, this technique in itself is rarely diagnostic and its results are

often interpreted in the context of data provided by other diagnostic procedures

may be used for suspected Sjögren's syndrome or chronic sialadenitis – in the latter case to determine whether the gland requires surgical extirpation.

MINOR ORAL SURGERY AND SALIVARY GLAND DISEASE

A senior house officer in oral and maxillofacial surgery at a general hospital may participate in the diagnosis and management of salivary gland disease in the following ways.

Diagnosis

- **Biopsy for suspected Sjögren's syndrome:**
  minor salivary glands of the lower lip are the most common biopsy tissue procured for diagnosis of Sjögren's syndrome
  the technique is performed under local anaesthesia
  paramedian vertical incision of lower labial mucosa
  blunt submucous dissection and stretching the incision site allows minor salivary glands to appear prominently through the incision
  minimum of five lobules of minor salivary glands required for pathological examination
  haemostasis and primary closure of labial incision.
- **Biopsy for suspected tumours of intraoral glands:**
  incisional biopsy may be obtained by a small incision along the mucosa and procurement of a piece of salivary tissue in the submucosa together with an ellipse of overlying mucosa
  whenever possible, biopsy the central part of the lesion, since peripheral biopsies may risk seeding of neoplastic tissues into peripheral tissues making it difficult to obtain a clear margin during subsequent definitive surgery
  haemostasis is followed by primary closure with a non-resorbable suture which acts as a marker of the initial biopsy site for subsequent definitive surgery.
- **Fine needle aspiration:**
  useful for suspected neoplasms of major salivary glands
  less likely to cause tumour seeding than with more invasive biopsy techniques
  this technique is best performed by experienced surgeons or pathologists.

Treatment

A senior house officer in oral and maxillofacial surgery may be involved in the treatment of the following salivary gland disorder (Figures 12.6 and 12.7).

- **Mucoceles of the lower lip:**
  sagittal incision over the mucocele
  blunt dissection to expose the mucocele

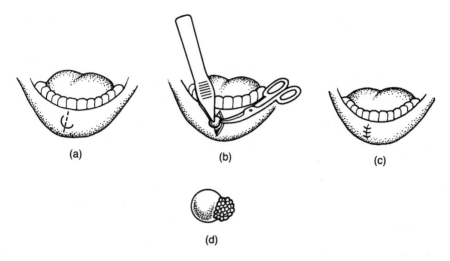

Figure 12.6 Excision of mucocele from lower lip: a, vertical incision; b, sharp dissection of mucocele from surrounding tissues; c, primary closure; d, associated minor salivary glands must also be removed together with the mucocele.

excision of the mucocele together with associated minor salivary gland

primary closure with 4/0 or 5/0 resorbable interrupted sutures

complications – wound dehiscence, recurrence, lip paraesthesia/anaesthesia.

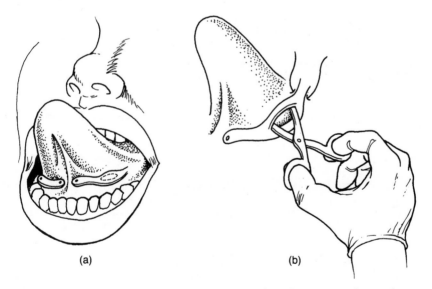

Figure 12.7 Removal of submandibular calculus or stone from duct: a, suture is passed behind the stone to prevent its posterior displacement during surgery; b, longitudinal incision is made along the duct and stone is further exposed by blunt dissection with mosquito forceps.

- **Removal of salivary calculi from the anterior part of the submandibular duct:**

    inferior dental nerve local anaesthesia, including the lingual nerve
    suture is passed behind the stone to prevent backward displacement
    longitudinal floor of mouth incision through mucosa only
    duct is identified and longitudinal incision made into the lumen of the duct directly over the stone
    stone is removed
    duct lumen is thoroughly irrigated
    incision in duct is left unsutured to avoid stricture
    floor of mouth incision is primarily closed with interrupted sutures.

Thermal surgery

Thermal surgery employs extremes of temperature as a means of tissue destruction. It is relatively conservative surgery with minimal morbidity which has a limited but useful role in the management of some small surgical pathology.

Cryosurgery

Cryosurgery employs subzero temperatures to destroy pathological tissue. Tissue destruction is achieved by:

1. Cryonecrosis – ice crystal formation in intracellular and extracellular compartments. Temperature must be at least $-15\,°C$ for cell death. It has been suggested that for malignant tumours $-50\,°C$ may be more appropriate.
2. Occlusion of microcirculation.
3. Stimulation of immune system through tissue damage.
4. Devitalization of bone, nerves and blood vessels, enabling the preservation of these structures as free grafts for subsequent cellular recolonization.

TECHNIQUE

- Liquid nitrogen may be applied directly to pathological tissues as a vapour or through a fine nozzle under high pressure.
- Two to four cycles of rapid cooling with gradual thawing are applied.

CLINICAL APPLICATIONS IN ORAL PATHOLOGY

Cryosurgery is suitable for:

    small vascular lesions – haemangiomas, vascular anomalies
    small areas of benign or dysplastic lesions of the oral mucosa; most effective with lesions overlying bone such as the palate or alveolar ridge.

LIMITATIONS

1. There is evidence that inadequate treatment of premalignant lesions with cryosurgery may promote rapid malignant change.
2. No tissue is available for histopathological examination.
3. There is no way of determining adequacy of margins and depth of tissue destruction.

Laser surgery

Laser beams are used in a sophisticated technique that employs temperatures over 100 °C to destroy pathological tissues by way of pure beams of light of various wavelengths focused at very high density.

CLINICAL APPLICATIONS

1. Destruction of cells – through vaporization.
2. Haemostasis – through heat coagulative necrosis.
3. Fine incisions.

CARBON DIOXIDE LASERS

Carbon dioxide lasers are the standard with which all other lasers are compared.

Initially, lesions were treated by vaporization. Current practice is to excise lesions so that tissue is available for histopathological diagnosis.

Carbon dioxide lasers are used for leukoplakia and small exophytic lesions. Neodymium–yttrium lasers are occasionally used where large blood vessels (up to 1.5 mm) are encountered and require coagulation.

COMPARISON WITH CONVENTIONAL SURGERY TECHNIQUES

- **Advantages:**
  cutting and destruction of lesion with minimal blood loss
  reduced postoperative deformity and scarring of surgical wound
  rapid healing
  reduction in postoperative pain.
- **Disadvantages:**
  expensive equipment and maintenance
  extra precautions necessary when using lasers, such as protective goggles, beam stops to protect adjacent tissues, special non-reflective retractors, and keeping flammable substances at a safe distance
  difficult to ascertain the adequacy of tumour removal (i.e. clear margins) owing to vaporization effects of laser on the margins of the tissue specimen.

Further reading

Bradley PF, ed. (1986) *Cryosurgery of the Maxillofacial Region*. Vols 1, 2. Florida: Boca Raton.

Cawson RA, Eveson JW (1987) *Oral Pathology and Diagnosis*. London: Heinemann.

Cawson RA, Odell EW (1993) *Oral Pathology*. Edinburgh: Churchill Livingstone.

Frame JW (1985) Removal of oral tissue pathology with CO_2 laser. *Br J Oral Maxillofac Surg*, **43**, 850–855.

Freedman PD, Jones AC (1994) A pathologist's approach to tissue diagnosis. In *Surgical pathology: considerations in diagnosis and management* (L. Gold, ed.). *Oral Maxillofac Surg Clinics North Am*, **6**, 357–375.

Gold L, Upton GW, Marx RE (1991) Standardized surgical terminology for the excision of lesions in bone: an argument for accuracy in reporting. *J Oral Maxillofac Surg*, **49**, 1214–1217.

Graamans K, van den Akker HP (1991) *Diagnosis of Salivary Gland Disorders*. Kluwer.

Howe GL (1985) *Minor Oral Surgery*. 3rd edn, pp 332–346. Oxford: Butterworth-Heinemann.

Peterson LJ, Ellis III E, Hupp JR, Tucker MR (1993) *Contemporary Oral and Maxillofacial Surgery*. 2nd edn, pp 526–555. St Louis: Mosby.

Shear M (1992) *Cysts of the Oral Region*. Oxford: Butterworth-Heinemann.

Soames JU, Southam JC (1992) *Oral Pathology*. 2nd edn. Oxford: Oxford Medical.

van der Waal I (1991) *Diseases of the Jaws: Diagnosis and Treatment*. Copenhagen: Munksgaard.

13 Postoperative care

Clear communication is the single most important ingredient in the administration of postoperative care. It is the clinician's duty to inform patients of what to expect after surgery and whom to contact if problems arise. Verbal instructions should always be reinforced with simple and clearly written postoperative instructions with emergency contact numbers for all patients who have undergone minor oral surgery. This is essential considering that verbal instructions alone are easily forgotten by patients who are often highly stressed by the surgery (Figure 13.1).

Instructions on postoperative care after minor oral surgery should include notes on the following:

1. Haemorrhage.
2. Oedema.
3. Nausea and vomiting.
4. Wound hygiene.
5. Rest.
6. Nutrition.
7. Smoking and alcohol.
8. Pain relief.

Haemorrhage

Complete haemostasis at the conclusion of surgery should be achieved before the patient is discharged. If there is persistent oozing, the patient must remain in the surgery until it stops spontaneously or measures are taken to effectively control it. Never discharge a patient with unchecked bleeding. (See also Chapter 14.)

There are three stages where persistent haemorrhage may appear.

Primary haemorrhage

When teeth have been extracted, the patient should bite on a clean gauze moistened with warm sterile saline if available, for about 20–30 minutes.

If bleeding persists after this time then further steps should be taken to arrest the bleeding, such as suturing or inserting a haemostatic agent (e.g. Gelfoam or Surgicel) into the bleeding socket and instructing the patient to bite on a moist, clean gauze for a further 20–30 minutes.

THE ROYAL DENTAL HOSPITAL OF MELBOURNE

Form 318

CARE OF MOUTH AFTER ORAL SURGERY

INSTRUCTIONS TO PATIENTS

1. Do not rinse your mouth for at least six (6) hours after extraction, do not disturb the blood clots by sucking or putting fingers in the mouth. Application of ice packs in the first four hours will help to reduce swelling.

2. You may eat and drink after removal of the pad, but hot substances, alcohol and smoking should be avoided for 24 hours.

3. Vigorous activity should be avoided for the remainder of the day.

4. Be careful not to bite the numbed cheek, lip or tongue.

5. There should be very little bleeding following surgery, but if this persists then again bite firmly on a gauze pad over the wound. If bleeding continues then contact the Royal Dental Hospital.

6. Following surgical procedures in the mouth there is local swelling which reaches a maximum in 2–3 days, after which it should subside gradually. Frequent hot or lukewarm water washes (½ teaspoon of salt to a 200ml. glass), will speed the reduction of the swelling, and should be commenced on the day following surgery and continued over the next 5 days.

7. Post-operative pain should not be severe. If present it should be controlled by the tablets prescribed for pain. When necessary the prescribed amount can be taken every four hours, but if pain persists, the patient should report to the Royal Dental Hospital.

8. It is most important to keep the mouth clean following an operation, and toothbrush and toothpaste should be used freely, in addition to mouth-washes.

9. Food and non-alcoholic fluids can be taken freely according to the patient's tolerance.

10. In cases of complication or severe bleeding, treatment is available at the hospital.
Each Week Day, including
Saturdays, Sundays & Public Holidays .... 9.00 a.m.–9.15 p.m.
Telephone No.: Working Hours   341 0212
After Normal Working Hours   341 0422

11. If bleeding is severe outside these hours obtain aid at your nearest Hospital Casualty Department.

Figure 13.1 Patient instructions on postoperative care.

Reactionary haemorrhage

Reactionary haemorrhage occurs within 24 hours after surgery. Patients should be discharged with a small supply of sterile gauze and instructions on how to use it in case of bleeding. Further instructions about minimizing the likelihood of postoperative bleeding should include the following:

1. Avoid smoking and alcohol, particularly in the first 48 hours after surgery.
2. Keep fingers and tongue away from the surgical site.
3. Avoid hot foods and liquids, especially in the first 24 hours after surgery.
4. Avoid vigorous exercise and stressful environments.
5. Sleep with head elevated on several pillows.

6. In the event of bleeding, tightly roll up the moistened clean gauze provided, place it over the extraction site and bite firmly for 30 minutes. If bleeding persists in spite of local measures then contact the surgery, the clinician on duty or the nearest hospital for further advice.

Secondary haemorrhage

Secondary haemorrhage occurs about 10 days after surgery and is often due to an infected surgical wound. Secondary haemorrhage can be avoided if the patient maintains a satisfactory level of oral hygiene (see below).

Oedema

Patients must be informed that facial swelling or oedema is a normal reaction of the body to oral surgery and the severity of the swelling will depend on the difficulty of the surgery. Measures used to minimize the degree of postoperative facial swelling may include:

- **Careful surgery** – delicate handling of tissues with minimal tissue damage.
- **Increased operator experience** – which results in reduced operating time.
- **Steroids** – see below.
- **NSAIDs** (non-steroidal anti-inflammatory drugs) – the anti-inflammatory properties of this class of drugs have failed to demonstrate any ability to reduce postoperative swelling.
- **Ice packs** applied to the face immediately after surgery theoretically help to reduce facial swelling by reducing blood flow and hence the inflammatory response in the vicinity of the surgical site.

Steroids

Intraoperative use of steroids may be useful in dampening the body's inflammatory response to surgical tissue damage, hence reducing the amount of tissue oedema which forms an integral part of the inflammatory reaction. Unfortunately, the degree of effectiveness of steroids has never been accurately measured, since clinical studies are difficult to standardize and compare, particularly in the absence of adequate controls. Nevertheless, subjective experiences with steroids appear to demonstrate a certain measure of clinically apparent reduction in maximum swelling.

Steroids are best reserved for difficult and prolonged surgical cases and should be commenced immediately before surgery and continued for no more than 24–48 hours so that adrenal-pituitary suppression does not occur.

- **Some suggested steroid regimens:**
    dexamethasone 4–8 mg IV intraoperatively, followed by 4 mg every 8 hours for 24 hours
    methylprednisolone 100 mg IV intraoperatively, followed by 50–100 mg every 6–8 hours for 24 hours.

Nausea and vomiting

Patients must be warned about the possibility of nausea and vomiting, particularly after procedures under general anaesthesia. Nausea and vomiting may arise from the following causes.

- **Narcotics** – the use of narcotic analgesics after surgery is a common cause of nausea and vomiting. If this does occur the analgesics should be changed immediately to NSAIDs alone (see below). Inpatients who are prescribed narcotics following oral surgical procedures must also have antiemetics such as metoclopramide (Maxolon) 10 mg IM 6-hourly or prochlorperazine (Stemetil) 12.5 mg IM every 6–8 hours routinely added to their drug chart.
- **Blood in the stomach** – swallowing blood during and after oral surgery is a relatively common occurrence and often leads to vomiting since the stomach lining has a poor tolerance to blood. If this occurs, patients need reassurance, and antacids or indigestion remedies may be useful in alleviating the symptoms.
- **Starvation** – patients who have been fasting prior to minor oral surgery under general anaesthesia may feel weak and nauseated after surgery owing to low blood sugar levels. Intravenous administration of fluids such as dextrose or Hartmann's solution during surgery under GA will help restore and maintain fluid, electrolyte and sugar balance, minimizing the likelihood of nausea and vomiting postoperatively.

Treatment

In patients with nausea and vomiting, it is extremely important to maintain adequate hydration by encouraging them to drink plenty of fluids. Flat lemonade will at least provide the patient with plenty of sugars for energy. If the vomiting is severe and the patient cannot tolerate oral fluids, the patient must be admitted to hospital and commenced on intravenous fluids such as normal saline 1000 ml 8-hourly alternating with 5% dextrose to restore sodium and chloride balance. The resultant metabolic alkalosis must also be corrected and the vomiting controlled with parenteral antiemetics.

Wound hygiene

The oral cavity is a haven for a multitude of micro-organisms, yet oral surgical wounds have no higher incidence of infection than surgical wounds on the skin. However, unlike surgical wounds outside the oral cavity, oral wounds cannot be isolated with a clean dressing and so remain exposed to the hazards of the bacteria-laden oral environment.

A clean wound is conducive to rapid healing, so the patient must be encouraged to maintain a high level of oral hygiene. Unfortunately, tissue swelling and postoperative pain make brushing almost impossible, so mouth rinses are the next best thing to maintain a relatively clean surgical site. Two types of mouth rinse are commonly prescribed after minor oral surgery:

- Salt-water mouthwashes are found to have a soothing effect on the surgical wound and help to promote rapid healing. They simply consist of a teaspoon of salt in half a glass of hot but not scalding water. The patient is instructed to rinse the mouth out for 2 minutes before spitting out the solution. This may be done three to six times daily.
- Antiseptic mouthwashes are specifically used to keep the surgical site clean. It is most important to rinse the mouth out immediately after every meal. Probably the most effective antiseptic is chlorhexidine 0.2% solution, held over the surgical site for up to 1 minute and then expectorated. If used for longer than a week, it may stain the teeth, so brushing should be introduced gradually as the pain and swelling subside.

It is important to note that vigorous mouth rinsing should commence no sooner than 8–12 hours after surgery, so as not to disturb the initial blood clot.

Rest

Surgery is a stressful experience that often places the patient in an exhausted state of mind and body. A fundamental part of the recovery process is rest, and this should be emphasized to patients. Rest entails forgoing normal duties, including domestic chores, until the postoperative symptoms of pain and swelling subside to a degree that does not hinder normal daily activity.

Exercise

Any level of exercise should be discouraged, particularly within the first 24 hours after minor oral surgery. Thereafter, only light exercise such as walking may be permitted. Vigorous exercise such as weight-lifting or rugby football is best avoided until at least 3–4 weeks after surgery.

Time off work

Whether the patient takes time off work or is excused from normal duties will depend on the difficulty and complexity of the surgery and also the type of work the patient is engaged in:

a manual labourer should be advised to take lighter duties or even a few days off work after surgical extractions
an office clerk with a simple tooth extraction (e.g. an erupted maxillary third molar) may safely return to work the same day as the surgery.

In most cases, a medical certificate which excuses the patient from normal duties for a prescribed period will be issued by the clinician who must determine what constitutes a reasonable period of recovery. A clinician's judgement must not be swayed by patient requests for time off work beyond the expected period for reasonable recovery, unless postoperative complications arise.

Nutrition

Adequate nutrition is another important part of the recovery process after surgery.

- **Benefits of adequate nutrition:**
  increases the body's immunity and resistance to infection
  improves wound healing
  reduces the risk of surgical complications.
- **Limitations of diet** – unfortunately, minor oral surgery often results in intraoral pain, swelling and trismus that compromises masticatory function and limits the consumption of solid foods. Diet in the days immediately after minor oral surgery is mainly confined to:
  naturally soft foods such as eggs or soup
  solid foods that are processed through a blender to break them up into manageable pieces that may be swallowed with minimal chewing
  where foods cannot be tolerated (especially in young children) adequate fluid intake is essential, so the patient is encouraged to drink as much as possible. Flat lemonade is useful as an energy source; however, fruit juices fortified with vitamins and minerals and milkshakes are preferable
  various feeding preparations can be obtained from the pharmacy when there is doubt about the adequacy of protein, carbohydrate, fat, vitamins and minerals in the existing diet.

Smoking and alcohol

Apart from the general health hazards associated with smoking and chronic alcohol intake, there is also an increased risk of postoperative complications. Smoking and alcohol consumption after minor oral surgery may cause the following:

1. Reduced healing potential of tissues – delayed healing of surgical wounds.
2. Increased potential for wound infection, e.g. dry sockets.
3. Increased potential for postoperative bleeding, especially in chronic alcoholism.
4. Decreased immune capacity.
5. Greater likelihood of respiratory complications, especially after oral surgery procedures under general anaesthesia.
6. Adverse drug interactions between alcohol and postoperative medications such as narcotic analgesics and antibiotics such as metronidazole.

Patients should therefore be advised to abstain from alcohol and smoking throughout the postoperative course of recovery, and particularly while taking medication. If the patient has the desire to stop smoking, a few weeks before surgery is an excellent time to do so.

Pain relief

Pain is a subjective phenomenon that is difficult to measure, and is dependent not only on the complexity of the surgery but also on the patient's individual response to pain. Pain relief after surgery is an essential part of postoperative care. It is an area of surgery that has been the subject of countless studies and published articles, and yet there continues to be an alarming measure of apathy amongst clinicians about the important distinction between pain relief and adequate pain control after surgery.

- **Selection** – in an outpatient dental setting, the clinician has a large range of oral analgesic preparations to choose from. The choice will depend on the following factors:
    patient tolerance of the medication
    history of allergy
    complexity of the surgery
    cost.
- **Prescription** – when prescribing analgesics, the 'take as required' philosophy tends to provide brief periods of relief but with more frequent pain cycles, decreased analgesic effectiveness and ultimately overuse and abuse of the medication. It is now a more acceptable practice for patients to take their analgesics at regular intervals (not 'as required') for a specified period of time, after which sufficient symptomatic relief is achieved so that analgesics are no longer required. Analgesics taken at regular intervals will reduce the likelihood of intolerable pain, improve postoperative comfort and promote a more rapid recovery.

Types of analgesics

In minor oral surgery practice there are two classes of analgesics that may be used for postoperative pain control.

NON-STEROIDAL ANTI-INFLAMMATORY DRUGS

By far the most commonly prescribed analgesics, non-steroidal anti-inflammatory drugs (NSAIDs) are effective for mild to moderate pain arising from inflammatory conditions of superficial tissues such as skin and mucosa, as well as joints. Ideal for minor oral surgery, the most commonly used drugs in this class are as follows.

Aspirin

Aspirin or acetylsalicylic acid is rapidly metabolized in the plasma and liver to salicylic acid which has a much longer half-life. It is extremely effective in acute pain of an inflammatory nature (including surgical pain), although it is more often used these days for long-term treatment of painful arthritic conditions and prophylaxis against vascular occlusive disease than for postoperative pain. In minor oral surgery aspirin has been largely superseded by other NSAIDs because of its gastric ulcerogenic propensity.

- Dose: 600 mg every 4–6 hours.

Paracetamol (acetaminophen)
Paracetamol is an active analine derivative that has become a popular alternative to aspirin with effective analgesic and antipyretic properties but with very weak anti-inflammatory activity. Unlike aspirin, it is safe for children, the elderly and in pregnancy (except in the first trimester) and does not interfere with platelet function or cause gastric irritation. In chronic high doses (> 4 g per day), however, it is hepatotoxic and caution is advised.

- Dose: 500 mg 1–2 tablets 4-hourly.

Ibuprofen
Ibuprofen is a propionic acid derivative that is slowly gaining popularity as a first-choice analgesic following minor oral surgery. The analgesic and anti-inflammatory effects are comparable with other NSAIDs but gastric irritation is less.

- Dose: 400–600 mg 8-hourly.

Other NSAIDs
Other NSAIDs such as indomethacin and naproxen are rarely used in minor oral surgery because of their longer half-lives which are best suited to the management of chronic inflammatory conditions rather than acute surgical pain. Diflunisal, on the other hand, is currently attracting interest among the dental community although its introduction to widespread use after minor oral surgery remains to be seen.

NARCOTICS

Opiate narcotics act on specific receptors in the central nervous system, conferring a central analgesic effect that, unlike NSAIDs, is not confined to pain arising from inflammatory processes. At usual clinical doses, narcotics are more effective in dampening the patient's emotional response to pain rather than eliminating the pain sensation itself. Patients will still report the presence of pain but they are better able to tolerate it after narcotic administration. Narcotics are particularly useful for severe pain arising from deep or visceral structures. In minor oral surgery, however, narcotics are often used in combination with NSAIDs in an outpatient setting, and are rarely prescribed alone. The most commonly prescribed oral narcotics are as follows:

- Codeine 30–60 mg every 4 hours.
- Dextropropoxyphene 50–100 mg every 4–6 hours.
- Oxycodone 5–10 mg every 6 hours.
- Hydrocodone 5–10 mg every 6 hours.

Side-effects
Side-effects of narcotic analgesics include:

nausea and vomiting
constipation
hypotension
respiratory depression
tolerance after 1 week of continuous use (i.e. must increase dose for same analgesic effect)
potential for abuse and addiction.

Note: patients on narcotic analgesics must be warned of potential drowsiness that may impair ability to drive or safely operate machinery.

COMPOUND ANALGESICS

Often a combination analgesic preparation of an NSAID with a narcotic will be prescribed for minor oral surgical procedures such as surgical extractions that may result in considerable postoperative pain. The idea of compound analgesics is that greater analgesia is achieved using smaller doses than would be required with one analgesic alone.

Preparations and dosages
- Aspirin 325 mg + codeine 30 mg 1–2 tablets every 4 hours.
- Paracetamol 500 mg + codeine 8 mg 1–2 tablets every 4 hours.
- Paracetamol 500 mg + codeine 30 mg 1–2 tablets every 4 hours.
- Paracetamol 500 mg + hydrocodone 5 mg 1–2 tablets every 4–6 hours.

INTRAOPERATIVE ANALGESICS

Maximum pain intensity occurs about 3 hours after surgery, so a useful technique is to commence analgesia intraoperatively so that it is fully effective immediately after surgery. This helps to reduce postoperative pain when the local anaesthetic wears off or when the patient wakes up after a general anaesthesia. The most effective technique for immediate postoperative pain control has been the intraoperative administration of long-acting local anaesthetic drugs which maintain complete anaesthesia of the local surgical site longer than 3 hours after surgery. Intraoperative narcotics and NSAIDs have been far less effective in this respect.

Technical
Bupivacaine (Marcain) 0.5% plain with or without adrenaline – 2 ml of solution is infiltrated in and around the surgical site intraoperatively. Effective analgesia lasts for about 8 hours, although some patients may be concerned about the prolonged numbness, particularly when the inferior alveolar nerve is blocked.

Further reading

Berwick JE, Lessin ME (1990) Effects of chlorhexidine gluconate oral rinse on the incidence of alveolar osteitis in mandibular third molar surgery. *J Oral Maxillofac Surg*, **48**, 444–448.

Gersema L, Baker K (1992) Use of corticosteroids in oral surgery. *J Oral Maxillofac Surg*, **50**, 270–277.

Jones JK, Triplett RG (1992) The relationship of cigarette smoking to impaired intraoral wound healing: a review of evidence and implications for patient care. *J Oral Maxillofac Surg*, **50**, 237–240.

Neupert EA, Lee JW, Philput B, Gordon JR (1992) Evaluation of dexamethasone for reduction of postsurgical sequelae of third molar removal. *J Oral Maxillofac Surg*, **50**, 1177–1183.

Peterson LJ, Ellis III E, Hupp JR, Tucker MR (1993) *Contemporary Oral and Maxillofacial Surgery*. 2nd edn, pp 261–268. St Louis: Mosby.

Seymour RA, Walton JG (1984) Pain control after third molar surgery. *Int J Oral Maxillofac Surg*, **13**, 457–485.

Walton JG, Thompson JW, Seymour RA (1994) *Textbook of Dental Pharmacology and Therapeutics*. 2nd edn. Oxford University Press.

14 Surgical complications

The practice of minor oral surgery will inevitably result in complications from time to time. Although complications are uncommon, the patient must always be informed about the potential for problems to arise as a result of surgery. In clinical practice there can never be a guarantee that problems will not occur, although the clinician must reassure the patient that every effort will be made to minimize the likelihood of things going wrong. Recognized complications should be promptly referred to a specialist or to hospital.

Terminology

Complications – any adverse, unplanned events that tend to increase the morbidity above what would be expected from a particular operative procedure under normal circumstances.

Sources of complications

Surgical complications may arise from either one or a combination of the following factors:

- **The patient** – particularly those who are medically compromised, leading to an increased likelihood of complications such as persistent haemorrhage or delayed healing (discussed in more detail in Chapter 15).
- **The clinician** – risks are directly dependent on:
    level of training
    skills and experience
    attitudes towards total patient care.
- **The surgical procedure** – risks depend on the:
    complexity of the procedure
    local anatomy of the surgical site:
        access
        proximity of important structures – nerves, blood vessels, etc.

Only the last source of complications (i.e. the surgical procedure) is discussed in this chapter.

Complications of minor oral surgery

As with all surgical procedures, complications can occur at each of three stages.

- **Before surgery** – inadequate surgical planning and poor case selection may trigger complications during the subsequent phases of treatment, for instance, a medically compromised patient who is a poor surgical risk which is not recognized by the clinician (e.g. haemophilia).
- **During surgery** – intraoperative complications are often related to poor technique or lack of operator experience. Sometimes it may be the awkward anatomy of the surgical site that can lead to longer than expected operating times.
- **After surgery:**
    early – in the days immediately following surgery, complications are generally of an acute nature, e.g. painful dry socket
    late – in the weeks or months following surgery, complications are usually of a chronic nature, e.g. actinomycosis.

General principles of management of complications

Before delving into the common types of complications encountered in minor oral surgery, it should be emphasized that common sense must prevail at all times in order to avoid turning a minor problem into a major disaster. The general way to manage complications is to consider the following principles.

Preparation

1. Take an adequate medical history (Chapter 2).
2. Identify high-risk patients and take the necessary precautionary measures.
3. Clear communication is essential:
    inform the patient of what to expect and the surgical risks involved (obtain consent – Chapter 2)
    provide the patient with written postoperative instructions (Chapter 13)
    make sure the patient has the appropriate contact numbers in event of an emergency.
4. Follow-up appointments – to monitor recovery and identify early warning signs of an impending complication.

Response

- Immediate recognition of a problem – in order to permit a change of plan before a complication occurs. *Example: tooth cannot be removed with the dental forceps so rather than risk fracturing the crown, a surgical approach should be considered (Chapter 5).*

- Premeditated contingency plan – in the event of a problem arising, an effective response must be quickly mounted to avoid complications that are more difficult to deal with at a later date. *Example: immediately replace extracted tooth with the attached fractured maxillary tuberosity of bone to avoid having to deal with an oroantral fistula at a later date (Chapter 10).*
- Ready access to specialist opinion and immediate referral.

Intraoperative complications

In the practice of minor oral surgery the most common complications that may occur during surgery are as follows:

1. Dental complications.
2. Soft tissue complications.
3. Bone complications.
4. Nerve complications.
5. Sinus complications.
6. Instrument breakage.

Dental complications

See also Chapter 5.

FRACTURES

- Crown – due to gross caries, excessive force or brittle tooth that has been endodontically treated.
- Root – due to abnormal morphology such as fine-curved apical root tips.
- Adjacent teeth or restorations in adjacent teeth (not intended for extraction) through the clumsy use of instruments.

Management

1. Take radiographs to check root pattern and position of remaining fragments.
2. Difficult teeth should be approached surgically with sectioning of crowns and roots.
3. Prescription of analgesics and possibly antibiotics and prompt referral to specialist for further management.
4. The risk of removing small root fragments of vital teeth must be balanced against the potential complications that may arise if they are left in situ.

DISPLACEMENT

Teeth or tooth fragments can be displaced into various tissue planes, potential spaces or cavities.

- **Maxillary teeth or tooth fragments:**
  superiorly into maxillary antrum (Chapter 10)
  laterally into buccal space
  posteriorly into temporal or infratemporal space.
- **Mandibular teeth or tooth fragments:**
  lingually into sublingual or submandibular space
  posteriorly into lateral pharyngeal space
  inferiorly into inferior dental canal.

Management

1. Stop the procedure immediately to prevent the tooth being displaced further into deeper tissues.
2. Take radiographs in at least two planes to determine the position of the displaced tooth.
3. Inform the patient.
4. Observe the patient for signs of inflammation, sensory disturbance or infection related to the displaced tooth.
5. Refer to specialist for:
   immediate removal if tooth is directly accessible in superficial tissues,
   or
   removal at a later date if tooth is displaced in deeper tissues, to allow fibrosis to occur around tooth in order to prevent further displacement during surgical retrieval.

Note: retrieval of the tooth may be greatly assisted by the use of fluoroscopy.

SWALLOWING OR ASPIRATION

Swallowing or aspiration of teeth is especially dangerous in patients placed in a supine position with an unprotected airway and who are semi-conscious (IV sedation) or unconscious (mask GA).

- **Swallowing** has no serious consequences as the tooth is readily excreted by the alimentary canal in a few days. Chest radiography is required to confirm that the tooth is in the alimentary canal rather than the lungs.
- **Aspiration** is a medical emergency and requires prompt attention. If the tooth is lodged in:
  upper airway – perform Heimlich manoeuvre with application of sudden forcible pressure under the xiphisternum. Urgent referral to an ear, nose and throat specialist is required for pharyngoscopic removal of tooth
  lower airway – chest X-ray is mandatory with referral to respiratory specialist for bronchoscopic removal of tooth.

Soft tissue complications

TRAUMA

Trauma to surrounding soft tissues may be caused by:

excessive retraction forces
slippage of powered handpieces
use of hot instruments straight out of the autoclave
leaning an instrument against a numb lip.

PRIMARY HAEMORRHAGE

Primary haemorrhage from surrounding gingival tissues may be persistent
in cases of:

- Excessive surgical trauma.
- Inflamed tissues – which are hyperaemic.
- Underlying bleeding diathesis of patient due to:
    drug therapy such as aspirin or warfarin
    deficiency such as haemophilia
    disease such as leukaemia.

Management

1. Adequate record of bleeding disorders (see Chapter 15).
2. Local haemostatic measures:
    direct pressure by biting on gauze for 20 minutes
    suturing
    Surgicel, Gelfoam, topical thrombin, etc.
    diathermy where available.

PROLAPSE OF BUCCAL FAT PAD

Prolapse of the buccal pad of fat is a nuisance as it herniates into the
operative field, obstructing the view and interfering with access for surgical
instruments.

Management
Replace the fat back into the cheek.

SURGICAL EMPHYSEMA

Emphysema describes the accumulation of air in tissues which in dental
surgery may be caused by:

    use of high-speed air turbine handpieces with the exhaust facing the
    surgical site
    increased intraoral pressure through sneezing, coughing or nose-blowing
    after minor oral surgery
    use of hydrogen peroxide in the surgical wound.

Management
Minor surgical emphysema crackles when palpated and usually resolves
with time. Extensive surgical emphysema may lead to infection if antibiotics are not prescribed.

Bone complications

HAEMORRHAGE

Bleeding vessels within bone may be controlled with:

bone wax
compression or crushing of bone with blunt instrument
packing the socket or bone defect with ribbon gauze soaked in adrenaline-containing local anaesthetic solution
plugging the area with mouldable dental compound or a stent
replacing the extracted tooth – especially in cases of significant haemorrhage caused by the disruption of a vascular lesion in close proximity to the extracted tooth.

FRACTURE OF MAXILLARY TUBEROSITY

Predisposing factors

- Lone standing maxillary molar in elderly patients.
- Ankylosed maxillary molars.
- Large and complex root patterns of maxillary molars.

Management

1. Replace fragment and splint with sutures or dental wires for 3–4 weeks then plan for surgical removal of tooth once tuberosity is fully healed, *or* remove fragment and close wound primarily with sutures.
2. Instruct patient to avoid nose-blowing (see later).

TEMPOROMANDIBULAR JOINT DISLOCATION

Predisposing factors

- Excessive force used to extract mandibular teeth without proper mandibular support.
- Lax joint ligaments – patient has a history of recurrent dislocations.
- Patients on medications that have extrapyramidal side-effects, e.g. phenothiazine major tranquillizers.

Management

1. Digital manipulation of mandible back into place, making sure thumbs are placed in the vestibule clear of the occlusal surfaces of the teeth (Figure 14.1).
2. The use of narcotic analgesia, diazepam or local anaesthesia into the joints may be helpful in relieving the muscle spasm and discomfort of reducing the dislocated mandible.

FRACTURE OF MANDIBLE

Fractures of the mandible are caused by:

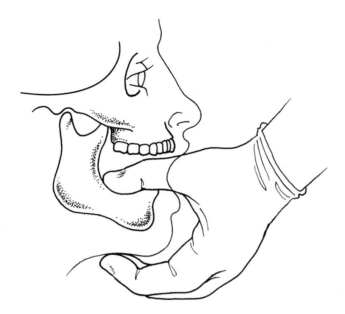

Figure 14.1 Reduction of a dislocated jaw: make sure that thumbs are placed along the vestibule and not over the occlusal surfaces of the teeth (after Howe).

excessive extraction forces on teeth in unsupported mandible
poor surgical technique – excessive bone removal.

Predisposing factors

- Buried tooth in otherwise edentulous atrophic mandible.
- Osteolytic pathology – cysts, destructive tumours.
- Brittle bone – osteogenesis imperfecta, osteopetrosis.

Management

1. Closed reduction – intermaxillary dental wire fixation.
2. Open reduction and internal fixation – *refer to specialist.*
3. Closed reduction with external pin fixation – in cases where pathology is involved.

Nerve complications

The inferior alveolar and lingual nerves are at most risk of damage from minor oral surgical procedures, particularly during lower third molar extractions.

LOCAL ANAESTHETIC BLOCKS

See Chapter 3.

- Direct trauma – penetration of needle into nerve trunk, resulting in a sudden 'electric shock' pain followed by deep anaesthesia.
- Indirect trauma – haematoma formed by direct penetration of nearby blood vessels by the needle.

Management

Explanation and reassurance to the patient is usually all that is required. The nerve will normally recover naturally over a few days.

LINGUAL NERVE DAMAGE

Lingual nerve damage may be caused by:

excessive retraction of lingual tissues
pressure from tongue retractor leaning against lingual alveolus
lingual split technique used to remove lower third molars
inadvertent severance of the nerve with a burr or scalpel.

INFERIOR ALVEOLAR NERVE DAMAGE

Inferior alveolar nerve damage, particularly in the region of the apices of the lower third molars, may occur in the following ways:

the roots may directly breach the inferior alveolar canal resulting in direct injury to the nerve upon removal of the tooth
upon attempted extraction, the root tip is displaced directly into the canal causing pressure injury of the nerve
inadvertent severance of the nerve with a burr.

MENTAL NERVE DAMAGE

Where the mental nerve emerges from the mental foramen, it is particularly vulnerable to injury from surgery around the lower premolar region due to:

excessive retraction on buccal flap
slippage of burr directly onto nerve bundle
apicectomy procedures on mandibular premolars.

GENERAL MANAGEMENT OF NERVE INJURIES

Review the patient to determine if sensation will improve with time. If there is no significant return of sensation within 6 weeks then prompt referral to a specialist is advised for nerve repair, which has the best prognosis if performed within 3 months of injury.

Maxillary sinus complications

Maxillary sinus complications (see Chapter 10) are particularly a concern whenever maxillary premolars and molars are being extracted.

BREACH OF SINUS FLOOR

An oroantral communication is created by the extraction of maxillary pre-molars or molars where:

the roots extend well beyond the sinus floor
the extraction is difficult and traumatic (e.g. curly root pattern)
there is a lone standing molar
the tooth is ankylosed
there is periapical pathology, e.g. a cyst or granuloma extending beyond the sinus floor.

Diagnosis
Bubbling through the extraction site occurs when the nose is blocked under pressure. The patient cannot suck through a straw or cigarette.

Management

- **Immediate treatment alternatives:**
   replace tooth and splint into position and plan to extract surgically at a later date, *or*
   cover defect with antiseptic-soaked ribbon gauze and remove in 2–3 weeks to allow healing by secondary intention, *or*
   reduce bony socket edge and suture margins together
   refer to specialist – who may opt for immediate closure with a buccal advancement flap provided the sinus is clear of infection.
- **Adjunctive measures:**
   instruct patient not to blow nose for 7–10 days
   analgesics
   antibiotics
   nasal decongestants and mucolytic agents
   if oroantral fistula does not completely close in 2–3 weeks then refer to specialist for formal surgical closure.

DISPLACEMENT OF TOOTH OR ROOT INTO SINUS

If the tooth or root fragment cannot be retrieved via the socket, then:

1. Stop the procedure immediately to prevent further displacement.
2. Take X-rays to confirm position of tooth or fragment.
3. Inform the patient.
4. Give analgesics, antibiotics and nasal decongestants.
5. Refer to specialist, who may elect to remove the tooth fragment either:
   directly, by surgically enlarging the socket and either suctioning or flushing out the fragment with saline, *or*
   indirectly, using the Caldwell–Luc approach via a surgical window through the anterior maxilla, giving the greatest access to the whole sinus interior.

SPECIAL PRECAUTIONS

Do not attempt to close a suspected oroantral communication when:

a tooth or root is displaced into the sinus
pus or purulent material is liberated upon extraction of a tooth
clear fluid flows from the sinus upon extraction of a tooth, which may
indicate the presence of a cyst or mucocele
unusual soft tissue prolapses through the extraction site.

This is mainly to allow free drainage of infection and necrotic material
from the sinus.

Instrument breakage

Needles and burrs are particularly likely to break. If the instrument is
easily accessible then remove it immediately. If it is displaced into deep
tissues, then:

1. Stop the procedure immediately.
2. Take X-rays to localize the instrument.
3. Inform the patient.
4. Give analgesics and antibiotics.
5. Refer to specialist for further management.

Postoperative complications

Alveolar osteitis

Otherwise known as 'dry socket'.
- **Classic presentation:**
    occurs about 3 days after extraction
    exquisitely painful, resulting in inability to eat
    very tender exposed bone where blood clot has broken down within
    the extraction socket.
- **Causes** – unknown. However, numerous factors have been implicated
    such as excessive surgical trauma, smoking, poor blood supply, infected
    blood clot which breaks down, etc.

MANAGEMENT

Local measures – under local anaesthesia the socket is irrigated with saline
to clear out the necrotic debris and a socket dressing is placed, which may
include anaesthetic and analgesic ingredients such as eugenol to soothe
the pain (Figure 14.2).
    Systemic analgesics are also helpful but antibiotics are rarely indicated.

Delayed wound healing

Delayed wound healing may be related to local or systemic factors.

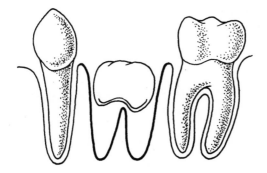

Figure 14.2 Dressing placed in a dry socket (after Howe).

- **Local factors:**
  infection (or rarely tumour)
  foreign body reaction (e.g. fragment of amalgam)
  poor oral hygiene – food and plaque accumulation
  poor compliance, e.g. patient continually picking at surgical site.
- **Systemic factors:**
  age – elderly patient
  drug therapy – e.g. steroids
  disease – e.g. diabetes mellitus
  deficiency – e.g. anaemia.

MANAGEMENT

1. Local debridement of wound with patient instructions on meticulous oral hygiene.
2. Where there is persistent delay in healing despite local measures, refer to patient's physician for further investigations of possible latent systemic disease.

Infections

See also Chapter 8.

- **Causes:**
  excessive trauma
  surgery on inflamed tissues
  general lack of resistance – e.g. in leukaemia
  haematoma formation – collection of blood in a potential tissue space which serves as a good culture medium for bacteria
  poor patient compliance – e.g. poor oral hygiene.

CLINICAL PRESENTATION

- **Local involvement:**
  pain, erythema, swelling, pus and fistula formation.

- **Systemic involvement:**
  increased temperature, pulse rate and respiration rate
  lymphadenopathy, malaise and increased white cell count.

MANAGEMENT

- **Local measures:**
  incise and drain fluctuant swelling, e.g. pus or haematoma
  maintain drainage, i.e. drain tubes or strips, warm salt-water mouth rinses
  debride necrotic tissue and irrigate area.
- **Systemic measures** (in conjunction with local treatment):
  rest, fluids and warmth
  analgesics
  antimicrobial chemotherapy (culture and sensitivity tests are ideal but not always clinically practical).

CHRONIC INFECTIONS

Chronic infections such as actinomycosis or osteomyelitis are rare after minor oral surgery and usually require referral for specialist attention.

Haemorrhage

DELAYED HAEMORRHAGE

Delayed haemorrhage occurs within 24–48 hours after surgery and may be due to increased blood flow to the surgical site as a hypertensive response to postoperative pain. On rare occasions it may be due to an undiagnosed bleeding diathesis such as von Willebrand's disease (Chapter 15).

SECONDARY HAEMORRHAGE

Secondary haemorrhage classically occurs about 10 days after surgery and is often caused by a breakdown in the blood clot owing to infection.

Management

1. Strong light and good suction to determine the site of bleeding.
2. Clean out surgical site with saline, then get patient to bite on gauze for 20–30 minutes.
3. If bleeding persists, consider further local measures such as suturing, or packing haemostatic agents such as Gelfoam or Surgicel into the bleeding site.
4. If bleeding persists despite local measures, refer to hospital for full haematological screening and management for possible underlying systemic bleeding disorder.

Necrosis of mucous membrane

- Possible causes:
    palatal injection under excessive force
    poor flap design – compromised blood supply due to excessive stretching, tearing or base too narrow (Chapter 5)
    poor aftercare of wound (Chapter 13)
    systemic disorders such as neutropenia.

MANAGEMENT

Local debridement of necrotic wound and meticulous toilet of area to allow healing by secondary intention.

Persistent pain

Pain that persists beyond the normal expected period for wound healing, in the absence of infection or delayed wound healing, may be the result of one of the following:

    traumatic neuroma
    causalgia (phantom tooth pain)
    psychogenic pain.

MANAGEMENT

1. Reassess original diagnosis – has the wrong tooth been extracted?
2. Establish an accurate history of the nature of the pain.
3. Eliminate the possibility of any physical causes for the pain such as co-existing disease (e.g. infected residual cyst).
4. Determine the response of the pain to local anaesthetic infiltrations and commonly used analgesics.
5. If pain continues for more than 2–3 weeks then refer to a specialist for further management.

Further reading

Alling III CC (1986) Dysesthesia of the lingual and inferior alveolar nerves following third molar surgery. *J Oral Maxillofac Surg*, **44**, 454.

Alling III CC, Helfrick JF, Alling RD (1993) *Impacted Teeth*, pp 353–369. Philadelphia: Saunders.

Goldberg MH, Nemarich AN, Marco WP (1985) Complications after mandibular third molar surgery: a statistical analysis of 500 consecutive procedures in private practice. *J Am Dent Assoc*, **111**, 277.

Krekmanov L, Nordenram A (1986) Postoperative complications after surgical removal of mandibular third molars. *Int J Oral Maxillofac Surg*, **15**, 25.

Larsen PE (1992) Alveolar osteitis after surgical removal of impacted third molars: identification of the patient risk. *O Surg O Med O Path*, **73**, 393–397.

Moore JR, Gillbe GV (1991) *Principles of Oral Surgery*. 4th edn, pp 113–128. Manchester University Press.

Oberman M, Horowitz I, Ramon Y (1986) Accidental displacement of impacted third molars. *Int J Oral Maxillofac Surg*, **15**, 756–758.

Peterson LJ, Ellis III E, Hupp JR, Tucker MR (1993) *Contemporary Oral and Maxillofacial Surgery*. 2nd edn, pp 269–288. St Louis: Mosby.

170Tetsch P, Wagner W (1985) *Operative Extraction of Wisdom Teeth*, pp 108–134. London: Wolfe.

15 The medically compromised patient

Advances in modern medicine have resulted in the improved survival of people with significant medical conditions. The growing number of medically compromised patients, particularly those with potentially life-threatening disease, have made it more than likely that such patients will present to a general dentist for minor oral surgery. Since medically compromised patients have a higher than normal risk of developing complications from minor oral surgery, the dentist must be able to recognize and deal with such cases in the safest possible manner. The aim of this chapter is to present only the most common disorders likely to be encountered in general dental practice.

Screening the medically compromised patient

In an ordinary dental office setting, it is unlikely that the dental surgeon will undertake a full physical examination prior to minor oral surgical procedures (see Chapter 17). Instead, the dentist must rely on a medical history to help identify patients with medical conditions that will require precautionary measures. All patients presenting for minor oral surgery must undergo a medical screening that involves a written questionnaire, which should include the following headings (see Chapter 2):

   allergies
   current medication
   illness and hospitalizations
   operations.

Any significant findings – e.g. allergy to penicillin – must be boldly recorded and highlighted on all patient treatment records.

The purpose of a medical history

A medical history allows precautionary measures to be taken that will ensure patient safety during minor oral surgery procedures. These measures may include:

1. Further investigations, e.g. clotting screen for those with a history of bleeding.

2. Alteration of the patient's current medication to facilitate the surgery, e.g. stopping warfarin preoperatively. This must only be done in consultation with the patient's physician.
3. The provision of preoperative medication:
     antibiotic cover
     steroid cover
     sedation.
4. Selection of an anaesthetic agent that is safe for the patient.
5. Undertaking the surgery in a hospital environment where appropriate medical back-up facilities exist (see Chapter 17).
6. Selection of postoperative medications such as antibiotics and analgesics that are safe for the patient to take, e.g. avoiding penicillins in those with a reported history of allergy.
7. Anticipating and preparing for a potential medical emergency (see Chapter 16).

Medical disorders in dental practice

A number of fairly common medical conditions have a significant impact on the way outpatient minor oral surgical procedures may be carried out. These conditions are listed below.

1. Pregnancy.
2. Cardiovascular diseases:
     infective endocarditis
     hypertension
     ischaemic heart disease
     thromboembolic disorders (anticoagulated patients).
3. Bleeding disorders (other than anticoagulated patients).
4. Respiratory diseases:
     bronchial asthma
     chronic obstructive airways disease (COAD).
5. Endocrine disorders:
     diabetes mellitus
     hyperthyroidism
     adrenal hypofunction.
6. Liver disease:
     chronic alcoholism
     viral hepatitis.
7. Acquired immune deficiency syndrome (AIDS).
8. Prosthetic joint replacements.
9. Morbid obesity.

There are also medical conditions where minor oral surgery is usually undertaken in hospital; these are discussed in Chapter 17.

Pregnancy

Pregnancy is an altered physiological state that entails important implications in patient care, treatment planning and surgical management.

OBSTETRIC COMPLICATIONS

Maternal

- Anaemia.
- Pre-eclampsia – a triad of hypertension, oedema and proteinuria.
- Eclampsia – seizures in addition to the above features of pre-eclampsia.
- Hypoxia – due to reduced oxygen reserve caused by raised diaphragm, increased metabolic rate and work of breathing.
- Disseminated intravascular coagulation (DIC).
- Thromboembolism – due to poor venous flow in lower extremities which may result in deep venous thrombosis (DVT).
- Morning sickness.

Fetal

- Fetal hypoxia – a major concern during any procedure or condition which compromises maternal respiration.
- Premature labour or abortion – incompletely understood although the following factors are important:
    severity of the surgical disease
    site of operation – sites remote from the uterus are less likely to cause problems
    anaesthetic technique – local anaesthesia is safer than general anaesthesia
- Teratogenic substances – drugs or X-rays. Effects of teratogenic substances include:
    before implantation (14 days) – death of the ovum
    from 14 to 60 days – period of organogenesis where major morphological defects may occur
    later gestation period – less severe morphological defects (e.g. cleft lip and palate), and functional impairment (e.g. reduced intellect).

MINOR ORAL SURGERY IN PREGNANT PATIENTS

1. Completely elective oral surgery is best postponed until 6 weeks post-partum, by which time maternal physiology will have returned to a pre-pregnant state.
2. Urgent procedures that can be delayed are best performed in the second trimeseter.
3. Emergency procedures for serious odontogenic infections should be performed at any time with caution.
4. Because of the risk of hypoxia, minor oral surgery is best performed with the pregnant patient in the upright position in the chair.
5. Although lead shielding minimizes the exposure to the fetus, elective dental X-rays should be avoided, especially during the first trimester of pregnancy.
6. Risk of DIC may lead to profuse bleeding after dental extractions which should be treated with local haemostatic agents (see Chapter 14 and below).

7. Avoid sedation and general anaesthesia wherever possible.
8. When using local anaesthesia, avoid prilocaine and felypressin (Octapressin).

DRUG ADMINISTRATION DURING PREGNANCY

Be wary of prescribing any drugs during pregnancy. Always consult a drug almanac when considering even the simplest of medications. Table 15.1 is a summary of the commonly prescribed drugs in dentistry and the relative safety of each class of medication when used during pregnancy. It is important to confirm the safety of the prescribed medication, including those that appear under the heading of 'safe', with a pharmacist.

Table 15.1 Relative safety of commonly prescribed drugs in pregnancy.

Type of drug	Safe	Unsafe
Antibiotics	Penicillins Cephalosporins Clindamycin	Erythromycin Tetracyclines Metronidazole Aminoglycosides
Analgesics	Ibuprofen Diflunisal Paracetamol (second and third trimesters)	Aspirin Narcotics Paracetamol (first trimester)
Local anaesthetics	Lignocaine Bupivacaine	Prilocaine
Sedatives and general anaesthetic agents	Ketamine	Nitrous oxide Benzodiazepines

Drugs contraindicated in pregnancy
Reported drug complications include:

1. Erythromycin (estolate salt) causes maternal hepatotoxicity.
2. Tetracycline causes hypoplasia and discolouration of teeth and bones in fetus.
3. Metronidazole is oncogenic in animals and increases the risk of midline clefts.
4. Aminoglycosides cause fetal ototoxicity and nephrotoxicity.
5. Aspirin is linked to oral clefts but data are incomplete.
6. Narcotics – chronic abuse results in fetal physical dependence, premature delivery and growth retardation.
7. Prilocaine – large doses can cause hypoxia in mother and fetus through methaemoglobinaemia.
8. Nitrous oxide inhibits vitamin B_{12} activity and increases incidence of spontaneous abortions.
9. Benzodiazepines are linked to orofacial clefts, cardiac defects and hernias.

Infective endocarditis

Infective endocarditis is an infection of the endocardial surfaces of the heart caused by bacteraemia. Endocardial damage, particularly of the heart valves, results from the formation of microbial vegetations which may also lead to emboli as parts of the vegetation break free into the circulation.

PREDISPOSING FACTORS

1. Congenital heart lesions.
2. Acquired heart lesions, e.g. rheumatic fever.
3. Turbulent blood flow, e.g. prosthetic heart valves.

CLINICAL FEATURES

1. Insidious, non-specific, flu-like symptoms: fever, anorexia, headache, fatigue, sweating.
2. Audible heart murmur.
3. Clubbing and splinter haemorrhages in fingernails.
4. Congestive cardiac failure – due to heart valve destruction.

ANTIBIOTIC PROPHYLAXIS IN INFECTIVE ENDOCARDITIS

Antibiotic prophylaxis is recommended for all dental procedures likely to cause bleeding. That means for all minor oral surgery!

Although infective endocarditis may be caused by many micro-organisms such as fungi, chlamydia and rickettsia, prophylaxis is mainly targeted against bacteria of dental origin likely to invade the blood stream during minor oral surgery.

- All prophylactic recommendations can only be considered as guidelines, for the following reasons:
    research into antibiotic prophylaxis has only been done in animal models
    retrospective human clinical trials have yielded extremely variable results
    an adequate human clinical trial may never be mounted in view of ethical restraints and the large numbers of patients required for the study.
- Statistical analysis suggests that the risk of anaphylaxis from prophylactic antibiotics is greater than the risk of developing infective endocarditis in all but high-risk patients.

HEART CONDITIONS NEEDING ANTIBIOTIC PROPHYLAXIS

The following list is based on the Australian Dental Association Guidelines, 1994.

- **Highly susceptible patients** (Figure 15.1):
    prosthetic heart valves

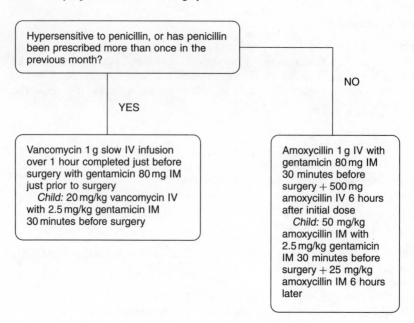

Figure 15.1 Antiobiotic prophylaxis for highly susceptible patients (from the Australian Dental Association Guidelines, 1994). Patient compliance is best for oral regimens and worst for parenteral regimens, so oral regimens should be selected where possible. Avoid intramuscular injections in patients receiving anticoagulants. A chlorhexidine 0.2% mouth rinse prior to oral surgery is a desirable additional step in antibiotic prophylaxis.

    history of infective endocarditis

    surgically constructed pulmonary–systemic shunts.

- **Susceptible patients** (Figure 15.2):

    most congenital heart conditions

    rheumatic and other valvular dysfunction, including surgically repaired valves and mitral valve prolapse with valvular regurgitation hypertrophic cardiomyopathy

    for 6 months following surgical repair without residual sutures or inserted material:

        secondary atrial septal defect

        ventricular septal defect

        patent ductus arteriosus.

Hypertension

Hypertension is the level of blood pressure that increases the mortality rate by 50% for a particular age group, i.e. over 160 mmHg systolic, 100 mmHg diastolic.

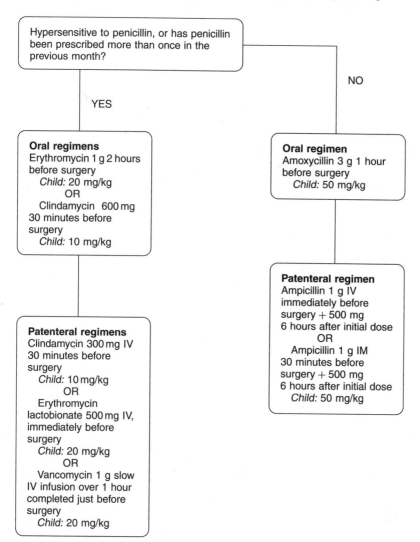

Figure 15.2 Antibiotic prophylaxis for susceptible patients (from the Australian Dental Association Guidelines, 1994).

CLASSIFICATION

- **Primary (essential) hypertension** – 80–90% of hypertensive patients are in this group, where no known cause can be identified.
- **Secondary hypertension** – 10–20% of patients are hypertensive because of underlying disease:
    renal – renal artery stenosis
    endocrine – thyrotoxicosis
    vascular – coarctation of the aorta
    gynaecological – eclampsia and pre-eclampsia of pregnancy.

COMPLICATIONS OF LONGSTANDING HYPERTENSION

1. Cerebrovascular accident – thrombosis or aneurysm.
2. Cardiac – heart failure or myocardial infarction.
3. Renal failure.
4. Retinopathy – papilloedema.
5. Headache – hypertensive encephalopathy.

MANAGEMENT OF ESSENTIAL HYPERTENSION

- **Non-drug measures** – weight reduction, decreased salt intake, stopping smoking, stress reduction, stopping oral contraceptive drugs.
- **Medication** – once commenced, drug therapy is continued for life. The following broad categories of medication may be used, sometimes in combinations depending on the patient's response:
    diuretics – for fluid overload, e.g. chlorothiazide
    beta-blockers – to dampen the sympathetic input that increases the activity of the heart, e.g. propranolol (Inderal)
    vasodilators – to decrease peripheral vascular resistance, e.g. hydralazine
    centrally acting drugs which compete with neurotransmitter chemicals of the sympathetic nervous system responsible for increased heart activity, thereby reducing sympathetic mediated increased heart activity, e.g. methyldopa (Aldomet).

MINOR ORAL SURGERY IN HYPERTENSIVE PATIENTS

1. Minimize stress levels – adjunctive sedation may be useful.
2. Avoid adrenaline-containing local anaesthetic solutions since adrenaline is a cardiac stimulant, although this may have little bearing on well-controlled hypertensive patients. Although adrenaline increases the systolic pressure, the mean arterial blood pressure remains virtually unaffected because the diastolic pressure is concomitantly reduced.
3. It is safer to perform surgery under local anaesthesia wherever possible, since general anaesthesia may evoke wild fluctuations in blood pressure that can be dangerous for the hypertensive patient. When general anaesthesia is planned, warn the anaesthetist, who may request further investigations and cessation of antihypertensive medication before surgery.
4. Primary and reactive bleeding from a surgical wound can be a problem where there is undiagnosed or poorly controlled hypertension.

Ischaemic heart disease

Ischaemic heart disease is the result of insufficient blood flow through the coronary arterie
s which supply the nutrients and oxygen essential for normal myocardial function.

MAJOR DISEASES

- Angina pectoris – chest pain, particularly on exertion, that is readily relieved by rest and nitroglycerine medication.
- Myocardial infarction – persistent and severe chest pain lasting longer than 30 minutes that is not relieved by rest or nitroglycerine medication. Referred to as a 'heart attack' by the general public.

PATHOGENESIS

In 95% of cases, insufficient perfusion of the coronary arteries is due to atherosclerosis. Atherosclerosis is the thickening of arterial walls with narrowing of the lumen which is caused by the focal accumulation of complex fibrous and fat deposits within the vessel walls.

- **Major risk factors:**
  hypercholesteraemia occurring below the age of 45 years
  hypertension occurring below the age of 45 years
  smoking
  diabetes.
- **Minor risk factors:**
  lack of exercise
  stressful 'type A' personality
  oral contraception
  obesity.

MINOR ORAL SURGERY IN PATIENTS WITH ISCHAEMIC HEART DISEASE

1. Minimize stress levels – adjunctive sedation may be useful.
2. Avoid adrenaline-containing local anaesthetic solutions, since adrenaline is a cardiac stimulant which may precipitate angina or cardiac arrest.
3. It is safer to perform surgery under local anaesthesia and sedation wherever possible, since general anaesthesia may evoke wild fluctuations in cardiac rhythm that can be dangerous for the patient with ischaemic heart disease. When a general anaesthesia is planned, warn the anaesthetist, who may request further investigations such as an electrocardiogram and chest X-ray prior to surgery.
4. Avoid elective surgery, especially under general anaesthesia, in patients who have had a myocardial infarct or coronary bypass surgery within the last 6 months.
5. Patients should bring their anti-angina medication with them and take a sublingual tablet immediately prior to surgery to minimize the cardiac symptoms that may arise from the stress of surgery.
6. Emergency procedures for cardiac arrest are dealt with in Chapter 16.
7. Some patients may be on low-dose aspirin which will create persistent bleeding from surgical wound. If aspirin therapy is not stopped at least 7–10 days prior to surgery, in consultation with the patient's physician, then strict attention to local haemostasis is warranted.

Thromboembolic disorders

Disorders of the circulation where there is an abnormal propensity for the formation of blood clots (thrombus) which move free in the circulation (embolus) to lodge at distant sites causing ischaemic damage to affected tissues supplied by the blocked artery. This section refers to patients on anticoagulant therapy.

- **Disorders predisposing to thromboembolism:**
  atrial fibrillation
  post myocardial infarction
  varicose veins in lower extremities – deep venous thrombosis
  carotid endarteritis
  infective endocarditis – heart valve disease.
- **Consequences of thromboembolic diseases:**
  stroke – cerebrovascular accident (cerebral embolism or thrombosis)
  transient ischaemic attacks
  pulmonary embolism
  claudication – lower extremities
  organ infarction – bowel, kidney or spleen.

MINOR ORAL SURGERY IN PATIENTS WITH THROMBOEMBOLIC DISORDERS

Patients are normally on oral anticoagulant therapy which will result in persistent bleeding following minor oral surgery procedures. When planning oral surgery, the dental surgeon must contact the patient's physician to discuss the possibility of stopping the anticoagulant therapy for some days prior to surgery. Such patients are best managed in hospital.

1. Patients on aspirin – aspirin affects platelet function for the life of the platelet, so therapy should be stopped at least 7–10 days prior to the planned surgery and recommenced 24 hours postoperatively.
2. Patients on warfarin (coumarin) therapy – the warfarin should be stopped at least 3 days prior to the planned surgery and recommenced on the day of surgery since it takes about 2 days for effective anticoagulant activity to be restored. An international normalized ratio (INR) test on the day of surgery is useful in deciding whether clotting activity has returned near enough to normal values to permit surgery. Ideally the value should be less than 2.0, although very minor procedures such as a single tooth extraction may be performed with values up to 2.5.
3. Patients whose condition is too unstable to cease anticoagulant therapy are best treated in hospital where they are given IV heparin until about an hour before oral surgery, recommencing about 6–8 hours after the procedure and continuing for 2 days until the oral warfarin regimen becomes effective again before being discharged.

Bleeding disorders

Healing after minor oral surgery begins with the formation of a blood clot in the wound. The development of a blood clot, or haemostasis, is a physiological process that results in the cessation of blood flow from damaged vessels. Haemostasis involves blood vessels, platelets and coagulation reactions. Disease, drugs or deficiency affecting any one of the three mechanisms involved in haemostasis will result in persistent postoperative bleeding that could be life-threatening for the patient.

CLASSIFICATION OF BLEEDING DISORDERS

Platelets

- **Decreased numbers** ($<40\,000/mm^3$):
  loss, e.g. massive haemorrhage
  destruction, e.g. idiopathic thrombocytopenic purpura (antiplatelet immunoglobulin G).
- **Decreased production:**
  deficiency, e.g. vitamin B_{12}, folic acid, aplastic anaemia
  disease, e.g. leukaemia
  destruction, e.g. radiation, cytotoxic drugs.
- **Dysfunction:**
  acquired, e.g. aspirin therapy
  hereditary, e.g. thrombasthenia

Blood vessels

- Congenital, e.g. hereditary haemorrhagic telangiectasia.
- Infections, e.g. septicaemia.
- Autoimmune, e.g. polyarteritis nodosa.
- Structural, e.g. scurvy (vitamin C deficiency).

Coagulation disorders

- **Congenital:**
  haemophilia A (factor VIII deficiency)
  haemophilia B (factor IX deficiency)
  von Willebrand's disease (factor VIII deficiency and platelet defect)
  rare factor deficiencies (I, II, V, VII, X, XI, XIII).
- **Acquired:**
  vitamin K deficiency
  liver disease
  anticoagulant medication, e.g. warfarin (see above)
  disseminated intravascular coagulation
  massive transfusion of stored blood (contains no viable platelets).

CLINICAL EVALUATION OF A PATIENT WITH A BLEEDING DISORDER

History

1. Family history of bleeding problems.
2. Prolonged or persistent bleeding following trivial trauma.
3. Medication, e.g. aspirin, warfarin.
4. Chronic liver, kidney or bowel disease – vitamin K deficiency.
5. Chronic alcoholism.

Clinical features

- **Platelet or vascular disorders:**
    more common in females than males
    persistent bleeding from superficial cuts
    petechiae – small red spots on skin.
- **Coagulation disorders:**
    more common in males than females
    ecchymosis (bruising)
    delayed bleeding from superficial cuts
    haemarthrosis – bleeding into joints.

Investigations

- **Full blood examination.**
- **Bleeding and coagulation times:**
    clotting time 5–11 minutes (simple test where venous blood is collected in glass test tube)
    KPTT 30–40 seconds (abnormal result indicates genetic or acquired disorders)
    PT 11–14 seconds (abnormal result indicates acquired disorder)
    TT 10–14 seconds (abnormal result indicates disorder in common pathway)
    INR (patient prothrombin time)/(control (normal) prothrombin time).
- **Special assays:**
    platelet function tests (aggregation with ristocetin)
    factor assays – VIII, IX, etc.
    fibrin degradation products
    fibrinogen levels.

MINOR ORAL SURGERY IN PATIENTS WITH BLEEDING DISORDERS

1. Identify the type of bleeding disorder with the help of the patient's physician.
2. Restore the haemostatic function of the patient prior to surgery by:
    stopping anticoagulant therapy (see above)
    replacement therapy, which should be arranged through a specialist haematologist or haematology unit. Replacement therapy is given according to the bleeding disorder and may consist of:
        fresh frozen plasma
        platelet concentrates
        cryoprecipitate (factor VIII)
        vitamin K
        prothrombin complex concentrates
        desmopressin (DDAVP).
3. Facilitate blood clot formation through the use of local haemostatic measures (see Chapter 14) such as:
    sutures
    electrocautery

local haemostatic agents, e.g. Gelfoam, Surgicel, fibrillar collagen, bone wax
warm, moist pressure packs.
4. Maintain the blood clot by delaying its breakdown with antifibrinolytic agents such as:
aminocaproic acid
tranexamic acid.

Bronchial asthma

Bronchial asthma is a reversible, paroxysmal narrowing of the bronchioles due to bronchial muscle contraction and swelling of the respiratory lining.

MINOR ORAL SURGERY IN ASTHMATIC PATIENTS

1. In the dental setting, an asthmatic attack can be triggered by stress or anxiety caused by a dental procedure, especially minor oral surgery.
2. It is recommended that asthmatic patients always bring their own inhaler along to every dental appointment. The patient is then able to take a prophylactic puff immediately before a stressful procedure such as minor oral surgery or during an acute attack.
3. Adrenaline-containing local anaesthetic solutions may be safely used, since beta-adrenergic receptors serve to reverse the effects of an asthmatic attack.

CLINICAL FEATURES OF AN ACUTE ASTHMATIC ATTACK IN THE DENTAL OFFICE

During an asthmatic attack, the patient will complain of shortness of breath (dyspnoea) and will want to be seated upright.

An audible wheeze (effort on expiration) with a tachycardia may resemble an anaphylactic reaction but without the facial swelling in severe attacks of asthma.

MANAGEMENT OF AN ACUTE ASTHMATIC ATTACK

1. Stop the surgical procedure and clear the oral cavity.
2. Seat the patient upright.
3. The patient should take two puffs on the inhaler (see above).
4. For severe attacks, administer the inhaler, give the patient oxygen and call for help (see Chapter 16).

Chronic obstructive airways disease

Chronic obstructive airways disease (COAD) is a general term used to describe a group of chronic respiratory disorders with a common pathology of compromised respiratory function resulting in decreased oxygen exchange and increased carbon dioxide retention. Examples include chronic bronchitis, emphysema and bronchiectasis.

MINOR ORAL SURGERY IN PATIENTS WITH COAD

1. Patients with COAD are best treated under local anaesthesia where possible and in the upright position in the dental chair.
2. Sedation and general anaesthesia should be avoided. If general anaesthesia is required for difficult surgical cases, then a full respiratory work-up is mandatory with the backup of a specialist respiratory unit.
3. Avoid administering oxygen unless the patient lapses into unconsciousness, since COAD patients are accustomed to low oxygen levels. More importantly, it is the carbon dioxide retention that acts as a stimulant for their respiratory drive. Therefore the provision of additional oxygen will only compromise their respiratory drive, resulting in apnoea.

Diabetes mellitus

Diabetes mellitus is characterized by an absolute or relative lack of biologically active insulin, resulting in a persistent state of hyperglycaemia (raised blood glucose levels). About 2% of the population are diabetic, of whom half are undiagnosed.

CLASSIFICATION

• Type 1 – insulin dependent diabetes mellitus (IDDM).
• Type 2 – non-insulin dependent diabetes mellitus (NIDDM):
      non-obese
      obese.

CLINICAL FEATURES

The clinical features of diabetes mellitus are summarized in Table 15.2.

INVESTIGATIONS

It is important for the dental surgeon to be familiar with the common tests for diabetes mellitus, particularly when confronted with a suspected but undiagnosed diabetic or poorly controlled diabetic patient. These tests include Dextrostix, random blood glucose measurements, glucose tolerance test, urinalysis, etc.

Table 15.2 Clinical features of diabetes mellitus.

Type 1	Type 2
Acute onset	Insidious onset
Young patients (< 25 years)	Mature (middle-aged to elderly) patients
Hereditary in 5–10% of cases	Hereditary in 90–95% of cases
Severe insulin deficiency	Normal (25%) or mild (75%) insulin deficiency
Thin	Obese
Shortened life-span	Normal life-span
Treated with insulin	Resistant to insulin

MINOR ORAL SURGERY IN A DIABETIC PATIENT

A dental surgeon performing outpatient minor oral surgery under local anaesthesia on a diabetic patient must consider the following precautions:

1. Adrenaline antagonizes the effects of insulin so theoretically it may be best to avoid using adrenaline-containing local anaesthetic solutions. In clinical practice, however, this precaution may be unnecessary considering the minute doses used.
2. Make sure the oral surgery procedure does not interfere with the patient's dietary intake and that the patient takes regular doses of insulin or hypoglycaemic medication.
3. Where the regular diet is to be disrupted by procedures such as preprosthetic surgery and the dentures need to be left out of the mouth during the healing process, then the onus is on the dental surgeon to provide advice on an appropriate soft diet.
4. If the planned surgery is expected to prevent adequate food intake then the patient is best managed in hospital (see Chapter 17).
5. Avoid operating on an uncontrolled or poorly controlled diabetic patient, since wound healing is usually suboptimal at the best of times and the risk of postoperative infection is significant.
6. Be prepared for a hypoglycaemic attack at all times (see Chapter 16), so have glucose readily available in the surgery.

Hyperthyroidism

Persistently high levels of thyroid hormone result in clinical features characteristic of hyperthyroidism or thyrotoxicosis.

CAUSES OF HYPERTHYROIDISM

1. Graves' disease.
2. Multinodular (toxic) goitre.
3. Adenoma (toxic).
4. Iatrogenic – excess thyroid supplement.
5. Follicular thyroid carcinoma.

CLINICAL FEATURES OF THYROTOXICOSIS

1. Weight loss with increased appetite and frequent defecation.
2. Dislike of hot weather.
3. Irritability, sweating and itching with fine tremor.
4. Exophthalmos – ophthalmoplegia with lag of eyelid.
5. Oedema in the pretibial region.
6. Tachycardia with atrial fibrillation at rest.

TREATMENT

1. Medical – carbimazole or radioiodine therapy if patient over 40 years old.
2. Surgical – subtotal thyroidectomy.

MINOR ORAL SURGERY ON PATIENTS WITH THYROTOXICOSIS

1. There is a theoretical risk of cardiac dysrhythmias with adrenaline-containing local anaesthetic solutions.
2. A thyroid crisis may be precipitated by infection or surgery, so beware and consult the patient's physician.
3. Minimize anxiety and hyperexcitability of the patient with the adjunctive use of sedation where possible.
4. Avoid general anaesthesia – may precipitate cardiac arrhythmias.
5. Patients with atrial fibrillation may be on oral anticoagulant therapy, which needs to be stopped and replaced prior to surgery (see above).

Adrenal hypofunction

The adrenal gland secretes cortisol and other important hormones. Adrenal hypofunction may result from disease, drugs or deficiency, leading to – among other things – inability of the individual to respond to stress.

CAUSES

- **Primary** (diseases of the adrenal gland):
  Addison's disease (autoimmune)
  tuberculosis of the adrenal gland
  metastatic cancer deposits in the adrenal gland.
- **Secondary** – adrenocorticotrophic hormone (ACTH) deficiency, hence decreased adrenal gland stimulation and secretion:
  prolonged corticosteroid therapy
  diseases of the pituitary gland or hypothalamus.

CLINICAL FEATURES

1. Weight loss, abdominal pain and diarrhoea.
2. Nausea and vomiting.
3. Weakness and debility.
4. Postural hypotension.
5. Hyperpigmentation – skin, buccal mucosa and palmar creases of the hand.

MINOR ORAL SURGERY IN PATIENTS WITH ADRENAL HYPOFUNCTION

1. Patients are unable to respond to the stress of surgery, trauma or general anaesthesia and may collapse (see Chapter 16).
2. Arrange a tetracosactrin (Synacthen) test if uncertain about adrenal gland status. The test is particularly useful for patients who have taken substantial steroid doses for longer than 2 weeks in the preceding 12 months:
   instramuscular injection of tetracosactrin
   plasma is collected before and 30 minutes after injection
   if the adrenal gland is functioning normally, the plasma cortisol level

Table 15.3 Steroid cover regimen for adrenal hypofunction.

Procedure	Regimen for patient who has taken steroids during previous 12 months	Regimen for patient currently taking steroids
Simple surgery (single tooth forceps extraction under LA)	Hydrocortisone 100 mg preoperatively – oral, IM or IV	Double current steroid dose preoperatively *or* Hydrocortisone 100 mg preoperatively – oral, IM or IV Continue normal steroid medication postoperatively
Difficult surgery (multiple extractions under GA)	Hydrocortisone: preoperatively 200 mg IV postoperatively 200 mg IM 6-hourly for 24 hours	Hydrocortisone: preoperatively 200 mg IV postoperatively 200 mg IM 6-hourly for 24 hours Continue normal steroid medication thereafter

If oral, give 2 hours before surgery. If parenteral, give 30 minutes before surgery. Monitor blood pressure throughout procedure.

will rise when challenged with the tetracosactrin, a synthetic equivalent of ACTH which stimulates adrenal gland secretion.
3. Prior to minor oral surgery, preoperative steroid cover should be arranged for patients with adrenal hypofunction (Table 15.3).

Chronic alcoholism

In chronic alcoholism repeated alcohol intake becomes detrimental to work or social life.

COMPLICATIONS OF CHRONIC ALCOHOLISM

- **Liver disease** (50% of alcoholics):
  fatty liver
  hepatitis
  cirrhosis.
- **Central nervous system disease:**
  Wernicke's encephalopathy
  Korsakoff's syndrome
  cortical atrophy
  fits and peripheral neuropathy.
- **Gastrointestinal disorders:**
  peptic ulcers and gastric erosions
  varices
  diarrhoea.
- **Heart disease:**
  cardiomyopathy.
- **Blood disorders:**
  macrocytic anaemia (vitamin B_{12} deficiency)

impaired host defences – protein deficiency results in reduced cellular immunity and depressed neutrophil function.

MINOR ORAL SURGERY IN CHRONIC ALCOHOLIC PATIENTS

1. Problems associated with alcoholism:
   aggressive behaviour and erratic attendance
   poor compliance with postoperative instructions
   dental neglect – advanced caries and periodontal disease
   anaemia – glossitis, angular cheilitis, aphthae and candidiasis
   increased bleeding tendency due to liver disease
   increased incidence of dry socket and osteomyelitis due to impaired host defences. Improved oral hygiene and nutritional support will help minimize this.
2. Drug interactions:
   general anaesthetic agents, sedatives and hypnotics all have an additive effect
   aspirin and other NSAIDs increase the likelihood of bleeding, particularly within the gastrointestinal tract
   metronidazole – nausea and vomiting when taken with alcohol.
3. Alcoholics are often heavy smokers, increasing the possibility of chronic obstructive airways disease and oral cancer.
4. Managing alcoholic patients in hospital – chlormethiazole should be prescribed to keep the patients from experiencing withdrawal symptoms during their stay.

Viral hepatitis

There are numerous viruses that infect the liver and cause damage to liver cells (hepatocytes) and compromise liver function. Some viral attacks, in particular hepatitis B, and C, may persist into a chronic phase leading to gradual erosion of hepatic function or simply carrier states that harbour the potential of spread to other individuals. The most common threat to the dental surgeon is hepatitis B.

PATHOLOGY OF HEPATITIS B

1. Caused by hepadnavirus (DNA).
2. Incubation period is 1–6 months (average 2.5 months).
3. Causes destruction of liver parenchyma and of virally infected hepatocytes by stimulation of the host immune system.
4. Over many months or years there may be:
   recovery – 90% of cases
   chronic hepatitis infection – with possible death in 5% of cases
   carrier state – 5% cases.

TRANSMISSION OF HEPATITIS B BETWEEN INDIVIDUALS

1. Parenteral – blood, serum (1×10^{-6} ml can infect).
2. Sexual – semen and vaginal secretions.

3. Maternal – in utero and through breast milk.
4. Saliva – lower risk than other routes.

IDENTIFYING HIGH-RISK PATIENTS

In dental practice, patients likely to have viral hepatitis may be identified by the following:

recent overseas travel – especially to countries where the disease is endemic
sexual practices – homosexual patients and prostitutes
history of infecting drug use – particularly where needles have been shared.

INVESTIGATIONS

When in doubt, tests can be ordered to determine the viral hepatitis status of the patient.

- **Hepatitis B surface antigen** (HBsAg):
    found in transient acute hepatitis B infection or persistent carriers of hepatitis B
    this test becomes positive 4–6 weeks prior to onset of clinical symptoms
    if the test is positive, then serum and other body fluids from these patients are infectious
    the most common first-line test ordered when there is concern about acute or chronic hepatitis B.
- **Antibody to HBsAg:**
    this test is positive in patients immune to hepatitis B such as those who have been successfully immunized or those who have recovered from acute hepatitis B infection
    most commonly used to determine if seroconversion has taken place following immunization.

MINOR ORAL SURGERY IN PATIENTS WITH HEPATITIS B

- **Cross-infection** when treating patients with hepatitis B can have dire consequences, particularly during minor oral surgery procedures. See section on infection control in Chapter 1.
- **Prevention** – all staff exposed to blood and other secretions should be immunized against hepatitis B. The vaccine consists of three intra-muscular doses of purified HBsAg from the plasma of symptomless carriers or a genetically engineered vaccine, taken at 6 weeks and 6 months after the initial dose.
- **Accidental exposure** (such as a prick from a contaminated needle):
    the puncture site should be bled and thoroughly washed under a running tap for a few minutes
    topical antiseptic should be applied

immediately give an intramuscular dose of hepatitis B immuno-globulin, prepared from high titres of HBsAg antibodies from subjects recovered from the infection. Vaccinated subjects should check their immune status.

Acquired immunodeficiency syndrome

Acquired immunodeficiency syndrome (AIDS) is an infectious disease with an underlying cellular immune deficiency caused by the human immuno-deficiency virus (HIV).

PATHOLOGY

The syndrome is caused by the human immunodeficiency virus – a retro-virus (RNA). Viral genome is incorporated into the host genome via the reverse transcriptase enzyme, by which the RNA is converted to DNA. Using the host T-helper lymphocytes, viral replication takes place whereby further viral RNA is produced and secreted by the host cell. By using the T-helper lymphocyte for replication, the virus gradually kills off these cells, resulting in a decreased T-cell count.

With the decreased T-cell count, there is a marked increase in oppor-tunistic infections in the host, which reflects a defect in the host's cell-mediated immunity. Eventually the host dies from overwhelming infection, most commonly *Pneumocystis carinii* pneumonia (PCP).

TRANSMISSION OF HIV BETWEEN INDIVIDUALS

Virus is present in high concentrations in blood and semen, although it is rarely recovered from saliva, tears, breast milk and vaginal secretions. Spread of HIV may be via:

parenteral exposure to infected blood and blood products
sharing of intravenous needle between drug addicts
anal or vaginal intercourse
perinatally to infants born to infected mothers.

IDENTIFYING HIGH-RISK PATIENTS

Because of the variable incubation period of HIV – from a few months up to 6 years – the virus may spread widely within a community before the disease becomes apparent and precautions are taken. High-risk patients include those in the following broad categories:

homosexual and bisexual men
patients with a history of injecting drug use
heterosexual partners of the above
babies born to HIV-infected mothers
haemophiliac patients and other blood transfusion recipients – particu-larly those who received blood prior to the introduction of widespread blood testing for HIV in the 1980s.

MINOR ORAL SURGERY IN PATIENTS WITH HIV INFECTION

- **Special precautions** must always be taken to avoid cross-infection during surgery (see Chapter 1). This must be done for *all* cases, regardless of whether the patient is in a high-risk category for AIDS or not, since in some instances asymptomatic patients may be unaware of or otherwise concealing their disease.
- **Surgery** – consideration should be given to providing prophylactic antibiotics for minor oral surgery because of the depressed immune defences often found in AIDS patients. Defer elective surgery when the T-cell count is low.
- **Vaccination** – as yet no effective vaccination against HIV infection is available for staff.
- **Accidental exposure** (such as a prick from a contaminated needle):
    the puncture site should be bled and thoroughly washed under a running tap for a few minutes
    topical antiseptic should be applied
    seek HIV testing within the first week of exposure and then again at 6 months
    seek counselling
    treatment – as yet there is no known cure for AIDS although the drug zidovudine (azidothymidine, AZT) has proved to be useful.

Prosthetic joint replacements

Patients with prosthetic joint replacements, in particular total hip prostheses, may succumb to infections that can result in the destruction and subsequent removal of the prosthetic joint. Such infections can be caused by bacteraemia that may arise from the oral cavity, particularly during minor oral surgical procedures. It has therefore been suggested that antibiotic prophylaxis should be provided for all oral surgical procedures undertaken in patients with prosthetic joint replacements.

CONTROVERSIES OVER ANTIBIOTIC PROPHYLAXIS

There has been no documented case of infection of a total joint prosthesis as a result of dental manipulations. There are, however, cases where infections of odontogenic origin have been reported, although not as a result of surgery.

There seems to be no convincing case that the complications associated with antibiotic prophylaxis outweigh the benefits of protecting against the theoretical risk of prosthetic joint infection.

It appears that antibiotic cover may be justified in certain immunologically compromised patients with prosthetic joints.

ANTIBIOTIC PROPHYLAXIS FOR PROSTHETIC JOINTS

1. Examination of the evidence reveals that for the majority of patients with artificial joints, routine antibiotic cover is not justified.

2. The dental surgeon contemplating minor oral surgery on patients with prosthetic joints must always inform the patient's orthopaedic surgeon. The decision to provide antibiotic cover prior to minor oral surgery should ultimately rest with the orthopaedic surgeon.
3. Where antibiotic prophylaxis is requested by the orthopaedic surgeon, the dental surgeon may employ the same antibiotic cover regimen as used for patients with infective endocarditis (see above).
4. It has been suggested that cephalosporin 1 g orally 1 hour before surgery may be a useful alternative to the infective endocarditis regimen, although, as mentioned previously, all regimens are at best only guidelines.

Morbid obesity

The morbidly obese patient is one whose weight is 30% or more above the average weight of the general population for their height and sex.

PROBLEMS WITH MORBID OBESITY

A morbidly obese patient may harbour one or more of the following diseases as a result of excessive body weight:

1. Hypertension.
2. Ischaemic heart disease.
3. Reduced respiratory reserve with laboured breathing.
4. Increased propensity to deep venous thrombosis.
5. Diabetes mellitus.

MINOR ORAL SURGERY IN A MORBIDLY OBESE PATIENT

1. The patient will be more comfortable in the upright position than lying flat during surgery.
2. Access to the surgical site in the oral cavity is difficult owing to enlarged cheeks.
3. Dosages of medication may have to be increased according to the weight of the patient for equipotent effects. However, caution must always be exercised, particularly when dosages exceed the normal safe limits.
4. Keep in mind the potential underlying diseases when operating on morbidly obese patients.
5. Postoperative healing may be delayed, with increased risk of infection – particularly in patients with diabetes mellitus.

Further reading

Field EA, Martin MV (1991) Prophylactic antibiotics for patients with artificial joints undergoing oral and dental surgery: necessary or not? *Br J Oral Maxillofac Surg*, **29**, 341–346.
Greenspan D, Greenspan J, Pindborg JJ, Schiodt M (1990) *AIDS and the Mouth*. Copenhagen: Munksgaard.

Hope RA, Longmore JM, Hodgetts TJ, Ramrakha PS (1994) *Oxford Handbook of Clinical Medicine*. 3rd edn. Oxford University Press.

Johnson WT, Leary JM (1988) Management of dental patients with bleeding disorders: review and update. *O Surg O Med O Path*, **66**, 297.

McCarthy FM (1989) *Essentials of Safe Dentistry for the Medically Compromised Patient*. Philadelphia: Saunders.

Porter SR, Scully C (1994) HIV: the surgeon's perspective. I. Update of pathogenesis, epidemiology and management and the risk of nosocomial transmission. *Br J Oral Maxillofac Surg*, **32**, 222–230.

Rose LF, Kaye D (1990) *Internal Medicine for Dentistry*. 2nd edn. St Louis: Mosby.

Scully C (1989) *Patient Care – A Dental Surgeon's Guide*. London: British Dental Journal.

Scully C, Cawson RA (1994) *Medical Problems in Dentistry*. 3rd edn. Oxford: Butterworth-Heinemann.

Stephensen E, Haug RH, Murphy TA (1995) Management of the diabetic oral and maxillofacial surgery patient. *J Oral Maxillofac Surg*, **53**, 175–182.

Woods R (1994) Antibiotic prophylaxis for infective endocarditis. *Int Dent J*, **44**, 215–222.

16 Collapse and resuscitation

Medical emergencies are fortunately uncommon in clinical dental practice. In spite of this, the dental practitioner must always be prepared to handle at least the most common emergencies that may occur in the dental surgery. Dental procedures are often stressful to patients and may precipitate a medical crisis that will require urgent and immediate attention in order to avert a major disaster such as permanent disability or even death. The purpose of this chapter is to familiarize the reader with the management of a collapsed patient in the dental surgery.

Terminology

Collapse – sudden loss of consciousness.
Resuscitation – measures undertaken to maintain life in a collapsed patient.

General management of a collapsed patient

Management may be divided into three main areas: prevention, preparation and treatment.

Prevention

- Take an adequate medical history.
- Identify high-risk patients:
     medically compromised, e.g. diabetic patients
     extremely nervous but otherwise fit, young and healthy patients

Preparation

- **Staff training:**
     all staff should be trained in basic life support techniques (Figure 16.1)
     life support skills should be maintained through regular attendance at continuing education courses.
- **Emergency contact numbers** must be accessible at all times.
- **Equipment:**
     availability of oxygen source and high-powered suction
     useful emergency kit.

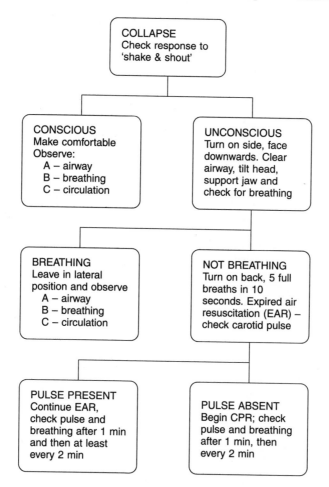

Figure 16.1 Basic life support flow diagram. CPR, cardiopulmonary resuscitation; EAR, expired air resuscitation.

- **Emergency protocol** – assign roles to each staff member to avoid confusion and delays in times of crisis.

Treatment

1. Prompt recognition of the early warning signs of an impending collapse is vital.
2. Act immediately – time is of the essence.
3. Always remain with the patient and call for help.
4. Lay the patient flat – trying to lift the patient out of the dental chair to place on the floor can be very difficult, with the risk of further injury.
5. Clear and maintain airway and provide oxygen if available.

6. Check for breathing and feel for pulse – if absent be prepared to begin cardiopulmonary resuscitation (CPR).

Note: correctly performed CPR is always better than clumsy attempts to administer oxygen or drugs that may result in unnecessary and dangerous delays.

Cardiopulmonary resuscitation

Components

- **Expired air resuscitation** (Figure 16.2):
    adults – 12 ventilations per minute
    children – 20 ventilations per minute.
- **External cardiac compression** (Figure 16.3):
    adult – two hands on lower half of sternum, 60 compressions per minute at 40–50 mm depth
    child (up to 8 years old) – one hand on middle of sternum, 80 compressions per minute at 25 mm depth.

Ratio of ventilations to compressions

ONE RESUSCITATOR

- **Two ventilations to 15 compressions**
    adult – 1 cycle every 15 seconds
    child – 1 cycle every 10 seconds.

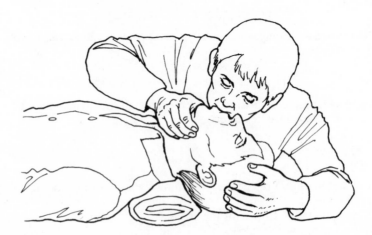

Figure 16.2 Ventilating an unconscious patient with expired air respiration. Note the head tilt, mandibular support and the pillow placed beneath the shoulders which are all essential in providing an unimpeded airway.

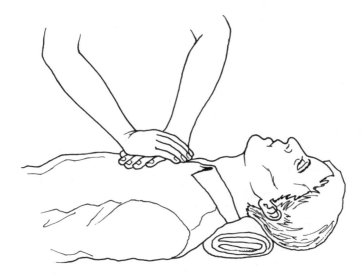

Figure 16.3 External cardiac compression. Note the position of both hands over the sternum midway between the manubrium and the xiphisternal process.

TWO RESUSCITATORS

● **One ventilation to 5 compressions**
  adult – 12 times per minute
  child – 20 times per minute.

Important points about CPR

1. Correctly performed external cardiac compression provides only 30–50% of normal blood flow to the brain, which is sufficient to maintain life and prevent brain damage.
2. There is no margin for inefficiency when performing CPR so practice is important.
3. If performed properly, CPR can maintain life indefinitely until expert help arrives.

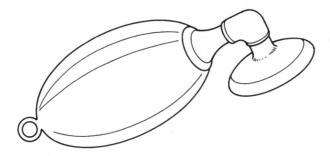

Figure 16.4 Air viva bag: a safer and more effective alternative to direct mouth-to-mouth resuscitation. An essential piece of equipment for all dental practices.

Collapse in the dental surgery

The most common causes of collapse in the dental surgery are:

1. Fainting.
2. Hypoglycaemia.
3. Fits.
4. Cardiac arrest.
5. Adrenal crisis.
6. Anaphylactic shock.

Proper management is facilitated by the ability to recognize the cause of the collapse. Hence the dental practitioner should become familiar with the clinical features that differentiate one cause of collapse from another. This will enable additional measures to be used to promote a more rapid and complete recovery.

Fainting

Fainting or vasovagal syncope is a transient loss of consciousness caused by decreased blood flow to the brain. This is by far the most common cause of collapse in the dental surgery.

- **Precipitating factors:**
    pain, fear, emotion
    postural hypotension – drugs, prolonged standing, etc.
    excessive heat.
- **Early warning signs:**
    pallor
    restlessness
    sweating
    sighing
    cold hands
    nausea and vomiting.
- **Late signs:**
    loss of consciousness
    depressed breathing
    brief convulsive movements
    cardiorespiratory arrest – death.

MANAGEMENT

1. Supine position – lay the patient flat with the feet raised above the level of the head, and recovery is often rapid.
2. If vomiting occurs the patient should be placed on their side to prevent aspiration.

Hypoglycaemia

Hypoglycaemia is a state of low blood glucose level which usually occurs in a *known* diabetic patient (see Chapter 15) and is caused by:

insulin overdose
missed meal
exercise or stress
combination of the above.

- **Clinical features:**
  rapid onset
  pallor
  sweating
  rapid full pulse – tachycardia
  intoxicated appearance – disorientation, irritability, aggression
  fits
  collapse.

MANAGEMENT

- If patient is conscious – give glucose orally in any available form.
- If patient is unconscious:
  protect airway
  place in lateral or recovery position.

From the emergency kit
Give glucagon 1 mg IM
or
Establish IV access – give 50 ml of 20–50% dextrose solution.

NEVER give insulin to a collapsed diabetic patient.

Fits

Fits may be precipitated in known epileptic patients by:

starvation
flickering lights
alcohol
menstruation
fainting
certain drugs, e.g. methohexitone (an anaesthetic induction agent).

- **Clinical features:**
  prodromal aura – patient can sense a fit about to occur
  sudden loss of consciousness (collapse)
  rigid extended appearance
  generalized jerking movements
  urine incontinence
  slow recovery with sleepy and dazed appearance.

MANAGEMENT

1. Remove obstacles from the patient's vicinity that may cause bodily injury during the fit.

2. After the fit, place patient in the recovery position and maintain clear airway until the full return of consciousness.

From the emergency kit

In rare situations there may be continuous seizures (status epilepticus) which may result in permanent brain damage or death if allowed to continue for 20 minutes or more. This must be treated with 10–20 mg of intravenous diazepam to abort the fits.

Cardiac arrest

Collapse from cardiac arrest may be due to:

- **Primary cardiac failure:**
  e.g. acute myocardial infarct (AMI) – cardiac muscle death caused by occlusion or insufficient blood flow through the coronary arteries.
- **Primary respiratory failure:**
  obstruction of airway – aspiration of teeth, vomit, etc.
  respiratory depression – drug toxicity or overdose.

HIGH-RISK PATIENTS

Patients most at risk from cardiac arrest in a dental surgery are those with a history of:

hypertension
unstable angina
previous AMI – especially within the last 6 months.

CLINICAL FEATURES

- **Symptoms:**
  central chest pain:
    lasting more than 30 minutes
    not relieved by nitrate medication, e.g. glyceryl trinitrate
    radiating to neck, jaws and arms
  anxiety
  breathlessness
  nausea and vomiting.
- **Signs:**
  cold, clammy hands
  distressed patient with ashen-grey appearance
  increased pulse rate – tachycardia
  cyanosis – patient turning blue
  feverish – temperature over 38.5 °C
  dilated pupils
  collapse
  no carotid pulse, heart or breath sounds.

MANAGEMENT

Irreversible brain damage occurs after 3 minutes so *act quickly*.
   Call for help and commence cardiopulmonary resuscitation (see above).

Adrenal crisis

The patient is unable to respond to the stress of:

   trauma
   surgery
   general anaesthesia
   infection.

This is due to the inability of the adrenal gland to secrete the chemicals
(adrenaline and noradrenaline) necessary to sustain the heightened level of
physiological activity required in such circumstances.

HIGH-RISK PATIENTS

Patients most at risk from an adrenal crisis are:

   those with a history of steroid use (more than 2 weeks) in the preceding
   12 months
   those with defective adrenal glands owing to disease, drugs or deficiency,
   e.g. Addison's disease.

CLINICAL FEATURES

1. Pallor.
2. Rapid, weak pulse.
3. Sudden and profound drop in blood pressure.
4. Collapse.

MANAGEMENT

1. Place patient in supine position with the legs elevated above the level of
   the head.
2. Monitor:
       A (airway)
       B (breathing)
       C (circulation).

From the emergency kit
Give hydrocortisone 200–500 mg IV.

Note: steroid cover is essential for patients at risk prior to any procedure
that may cause stress (see Chapter 15).

Anaphylactic shock

Anaphylactic shock is a potentially life-threatening allergic reaction to agents such as penicillin, or rarely to local anaesthetic agents.

- **Mild reactions:**
    sensation of warmth
    itching especially in axillae and groin
    feelings of anxiety and panic
    erythematous or urticarial rash
    oedema or swelling of face and neck.
- **Severe (life-threatening) reactions:**
    bronchospasm – wheezing
    laryngeal oedema – dyspnoea, stridor, aphonia, drooling
    hypotension – shock
    arrhythmias and cardiac arrest.

Note: any sudden and unexpected reaction to the administration of a drug should be suspected as anaphylactic since deterioration is often rapid.

MANAGEMENT

1. Stop administration of the causal agent.
2. Place patient in a recumbent position and elevate the lower limbs.
3. Check:
    A (airway)
    B (breathing)
    C (circulation).

From the emergency kit

1. Administer adrenaline 1 : 1000 (1 mg/ml) IM:
    adult 0.3–0.5 ml
    child 0.01 ml/kg
    this may be repeated at 5-minute intervals.
2. Administration of steroids, antihistamines and bronchodilators has a delayed effect and should not be used to the exclusion of adrenaline.

Medical emergency kit

Every dental practice should have a medical emergency kit. Although there are numerous emergency kits on the market, most clinicians prefer to assemble their own. It must be emphasized, however, that many components of a standard medical emergency kit require prior training in their use – for example:

    insertion of oral airways or endotracheal intubation (Figure 16.5)
    parenteral administration of drugs
    insertion of intravenous catheters or lines.

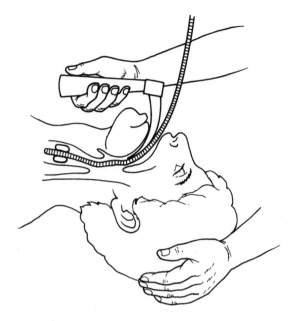

Figure 16.5 Endotracheal intubation using a laryngoscope. Note the head tilt and the endotracheal tube placement with the cuff inflated to seal off the trachea, thus avoiding air leaks as well as protecting the airway.

Components

A standard medical kit may contain:

- **Oral and nasal airways** – laryngoscope and endotracheal tubes (proper training is required in their use).
- **Syringes, needles, intravenous catheters and tourniquets** – for the parenteral administration of drugs.
- **Emergency drugs** – parenteral drugs may be preloaded at the appropriate dose into syringes. Always check expiry dates and maintain fresh stock at all times. Useful emergency drugs may include adrenaline, hydrocortisone, glucagon, glyceryl trinitrate, morphine, antihistamines and salbutamol inhalers.
- **Additional supplies:**
    glucose in powder or solution
    intravenous fluids such as dextrose and sterile water for mixing parenteral drugs.

Further reading

Brown AFT (1990) *Accident and Emergency Diagnosis and Management.* Oxford: Butterworth-Heinemann.

Evans TR (1990) *ABC of Resuscitation.* 2nd edn. London: BMJ Publishing.

Marsden AK (1989) Basic life support. *Br Med J*, **299**, 442.

Robinson R, Stott R (1989) *Medical Emergencies Diagnosis and Management.* 5th edn. Oxford: Butterworth-Heinemann.

17 Hospital practice

As a general dental practitioner the best place to acquire clinical experience in minor oral surgery is to spend a year or two as a house officer in the oral and maxillofacial surgery department of a general hospital. Being part of a large institution, the house officer or senior house officer has multiple responsibilities that ultimately ensure the effective day-to-day running of the unit. The aim of this chapter is to outline the role of an oral and maxillofacial surgery house officer in a general hospital.

Functions of an oral and maxillofacial surgery unit in a general hospital

In the complex environment of a general hospital, the oral surgery unit has a small but nonetheless important role as the sole provider of oral health care. These units provide a broad range of services as follows.

Accident and emergency care

The unit offers specialist and out-of-hours accident and emergency care, for instance a maxillofacial trauma service.

Elective surgery

- **Minor oral surgery:**
  under local anaesthesia and intravenous sedation – such as simple extractions. These simple procedures are usually reserved for medically compromised patients and emergency care for inpatients admitted for other ailments. In order to prevent a backlog of patients within the hospital system, simple minor oral surgery procedures in healthy patients are referred to outside practices
  under general anaesthesia – difficult minor oral surgery such as removal of impacted wisdom teeth is best performed in hospital rather than in a private dental office where emergency back-up facilities are limited.
- **Major oral and maxillofacial surgery:**
  routine procedures such as orthognathic surgery, temporomandibular joint surgery and removal of benign tumours
  advanced procedures – complex jaw reconstructive surgery, craniofacial surgery, head and neck malignancy – are confined to major centres having the required expertise.

Oral diagnosis

- The oral and maxillofacial surgery unit may be called upon to diagnose and treat oral manifestations in patients with systemic disease, e.g. oral candidiasis in AIDS patients, xerostomia in Sjögren's syndrome.
- Patients with isolated oral lesions may be directly referred to the oral and maxillofacial surgery unit for biopsy and definitive management.

Training

All oral and maxillofacial surgeons undertake the bulk of their clinical training within a general hospital, moving through the ranks of registrar and senior registrar until eventually appointed as a consultant.

Research

Oral and maxillofacial surgery units in many general hospitals undertake some clinical research, though often of minor significance. The serious research is usually confined to the major teaching hospitals attached to a university dental or medical school.

Visiting dentists

In some centres where there are provisions for visiting dentists, the following additional services may be provided under the umbrella of an oral and maxillofacial surgery unit.

1. The provision of emergency dental care for all inpatients in the hospital.
2. Routine dental care for patients whose medical conditions restrict them from receiving dental care outside the hospital.
3. Out-of-hours emergency care:
    odontogenic infections
    oral bleeding, e.g. after dental extraction
    oral pain, e.g. toothache.

Oral and maxillofacial surgery hospital posts

The house officer is usually a recent dental graduate who is employed by the hospital to carry out the day-to-day activities of running the unit. As such, the house officer has the most junior hospital position and is at the bottom of the pecking order behind the senior house officer (SHO), registrar, fellow, senior registrar (SR) all the way up to the consultant. It is the consultant who bears the ultimate responsibility for patient care, even though the registrars or senior registrars appear to make most of the day-to-day decisions on patient care.

Requirements of a successful house officer

The life of a house officer can be an arduous existence with tasks that range from mundane ward duties to seemingly overwhelming on-call commitments.

The following key elements are required to succeed in meeting the challenges of hospital practice as the most junior member of the team.

ORGANIZATION

A well-organized house officer will effectively maintain a tolerable workload and hence minimize the level of stress. Good organizational skills are essential for a happier and more productive working environment.

COMMUNICATION

In a large institution where the house officer must interact with senior colleagues, ward staff, other specialty units and the inevitable bureaucracy of administration, communication is an essential tool. The house officer must at all times maintain open channels of communication so that everyone – including the patients – is kept fully informed. Most importantly, the registrar must always be kept up-to-date with developments and events, no matter how mundane they may appear.

SELF-DISCIPLINE

The house officer must never be late for ward rounds, clinics, operating sessions or clinical meetings as these cannot function effectively without junior staff. If for some reason the house officer is held up in theatre or casualty, the SHO or registrar must be informed well in advance so that arrangements can be made either to relieve or to find a substitute for the junior staff member concerned. Drinking alcohol and fraternizing with hospital staff or patients while on duty are strictly prohibited and can be grounds for dismissal.

STRICT ATTENTION TO DETAIL

Nothing should be left to chance, and the house officer should always double-check that matters pertinent to the running of the unit are under control. Follow up any 'hiccups' in the system thoroughly and make sure all problems are being attended to before the consultant is called upon to make the final decisions.

Hospital practice

Hospital practice for junior staff entails the following responsibilities:

1. Admitting patients to the ward.
2. Preoperative preparation of patients.
3. Assisting senior colleagues in the operating theatre.

4. Ward duties.
5. Outpatient clinics.

Patient admissions

Admitting patients to the ward means that the hospital is taking responsibility for the patients' health and well-being during their entire stay in
hospital. It is prudent that the hospital, therefore, has an accurate and
detailed health profile of the patient in order to provide the most appropriate care.

ELECTIVE VERSUS EMERGENCY ADMISSION

Elective admission to hospital is a planned procedure that allows the
patient to become accustomed to the idea of a hospital stay. However, an
emergency admission to hospital is a frightening experience for most
patients, and this should always be borne in mind by the admitting clinician. Clear communication and a reassuring attitude are particularly
important for patients coming into hospital through the accident and emergency department.

ADMISSION PAPERWORK

Admission procedures can be laborious and are often left to the junior
staff. The house officer must quickly become familiar with the mountain
of paperwork and eventually cultivate a streamlined technique of admitting
patients to the ward, particularly when several patients are waiting to be
admitted.

ADMISSION PROCEDURE

The admission procedure consists of a verbal history and a complete physical examination (Figure 17.1). The house officer should consult the relevant
textbooks on this subject and observe admissions undertaken by more
experienced colleagues. Junior staff should never hesitate to consult more
experienced house officers or registrars whenever uncertainty arises or
abnormalities are picked up during the history or physical examination.

Verbal history

1. Presenting complaint – see Chapter 2.
2. History of presenting complaint – see Chapter 2.
3. Medical history – see Chapters 2 and 15.
4. Social history – see Chapters 2 and 15.
5. Systems history – the patient is systematically questioned about key
   symptoms that may be characteristic of diseases affecting various
   regions or systems of the body, as a guide to the subsequent physical
   examination:

HOSPITAL ADMISSION FORM   **DISTRICT GENERAL HOSPITAL**

PATIENT NAME.......... *Timothy Joseph Spencer* ....HOSP NO... *987654* ......
DATE OF ADMISSION.............. *14/5/96* ....

Chief Complaint.......... *Painful swelling in right submandibular region* ....

History of presenting complaint.......... *3 days and becoming progressively worse*

Medical   History
1.Allergies................ *Penicillin* ....
2. Current
medication.................... *None* ....
3. Serious illnesses
or   hospitalisations......... *Bronchial pneumonia 1993* ....
4.Previous
operations.................. *Tonsils & adenoids as a child* ....

Social History.......... *Alcoholic, homeless - 5yrs, no family, smoker >40 cigs day*

General Appearance.......... *Poor personal hygiene, smell of alcohol* ....
.... *Pale and mildly jaundiced* ....

Vital Signs.........BP.... *160/95* ..Temp.... *39.1'C* ..Pulse.... *85/min* ..Respir.... *15/min* ..

CHEST
    Heart - S1,S2. nil added, no murmurs
    Lungs - bilateral basal creps, central trachea

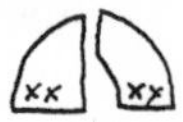

ABDOMEN
    Enlarged liver, lax, no tenderness, no masses, no scars 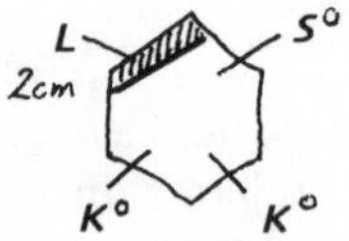

LIMBS
    peripheral pulses, clubbed nails

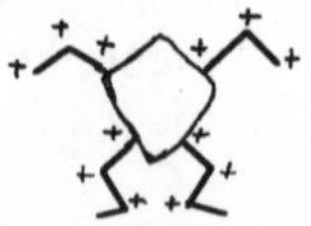

HEAD & NECK
    Cranial nerves 1->12 normal, fluctuant tender R. SM swelling.
    Oral airway patent, mild trismus approx 25 mm opening

ORAL & MAXILLOFACIAL
    Partly dentate, halitosis, advanced perio.
    Grossly carious right lower first molar (46). Tender to percussion

INVESTIGATIONS
    OPG - 5mm radiolucency surrounding apex of 46 distal root

DIAGNOSIS.......... *Acute dental abscess from non-vital 46* ....

SUMMARY   *49yo homeless male with history of chronic alcoholism
    presents with a 3 day history of increasing pain and
    swelling in the right submandibular region secondary to an
    acute dental abscess arising from a non-vital tooth (46)*

    SIGNATURE.......... *SHO - ORAL + MAXILLOFACIAL
    SURGERY.*

Figure 17.1 Example of a typical hospital admission record. Simple diagrams add a substantial amount of information to the admission record.

general – weakness, fatigue, lethargy, appetite, sleep disturbance, anxiety, stress, malaise

cardiovascular – chest pains, palpitations, breathlessness on walking or climbing stairs, breathless when lying flat, sleeps on multiple pillows

respiratory – dyspnoea, stridor, wheezing, cough (productive?), sputum (colour?)

gastrointestinal – abdominal or referred pain, diarrhoea, constipation, jaundice, colour and consistency of stools, vomiting, dyspepsia, swallowing difficulties

genitourinary – loin or groin pain, difficult or painful micturition, blood in urine, menstrual cycle

neurological – eyesight, hearing, altered sensation.

Physical examination

Establish a systematic approach to examining patients. Male house officers should always have a female chaperone present when physically examining female patients. The physical examination may be undertaken in the following order.

1. General appearance – thin, obese, pale, cyanotic, jaundice, anxious, alert, drowsy, withdrawn?
2. Vital signs – check blood pressure, pulse (radial) rhythm and rate, respiration rate, temperature.
3. Chest – assess heart and lungs:
    heart – jugular venous pressure, apex beat, precordial thrills
       auscultation – first and second heart sounds, additional heart sounds, heart murmurs (Figure 17.2)
    lungs – chest symmetry and expansion, tracheal position, percussion, tactile vocal fremitus
       auscultation – duration, pitch and quality of breath sounds such as bronchial, crepitations, rhonchi and frictional rubs.
4. Abdomen – observe distension, tenderness, guarding, scars of operation. Palpate liver, spleen and kidneys for size and position. Site, size, shape and consistency of other masses. Percussion, auscultation.
5. Limbs – peripheral pulses, fingers for signs of clubbing or peripheral cyanosis, skin lesions or arthritic changes, pitting oedema of ankles, palmar erythema, flapping tremor.
6. Head and neck – neck swellings, cranial nerve function I–XII, eyes (ophthalmoscope), ears (otoscope).
7. Maxillofacial region – the area of greatest interest is best kept until last. Check facial symmetry, patency of nasal airway, trismus, tongue colour (central cyanosis) and texture (smooth = anaemia), oral mucosa and teeth (see Chapter 2).

Preoperative preparation

Prior to surgery, the house officer must go through a checklist to ascertain that everything is in order and the operations can proceed.

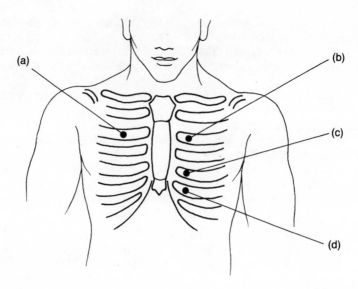

Figure 17.2 Standard positions for auscultation of heart sounds: a, aortic area; b, pulmonary area (second intercostal space); c, tricuspid area; d, mitral area (fifth intercostal space).

THINGS TO CHECK WELL IN ADVANCE

1. Availability of the operating theatre, the date and starting time.
2. The name of the consultant or operating surgeon.
3. The need for a preanaesthetic consultation for patients with special needs or medical conditions that will influence the anaesthetic management.
4. The need to contact the patient's physician or specialist medical unit for advice on management of the patient while in hospital. In some cases, the patient may need to be admitted under the care of a specialist medical unit (such as the endocrinology department for unstable or brittle diabetic patients) while in hospital for oral and maxillofacial surgery.
5. A list of patients (who have been contacted and are available on the proposed date) and the planned surgical procedures to be undertaken.
6. Prosthetic appliances and surgical stents have been constructed and are available in time for surgery.
7. A working diagnosis has been established from the results of special investigations such as radiology and histopathology.
8. Autologous blood supplies have been arranged for major elective surgery.

THINGS TO CHECK IMMEDIATELY PRIOR TO SURGERY

1. Admission of all patients to the ward.
2. Any additional results of further investigations such as special X-rays or blood tests.
3. Patients have fasted for an adequate period.
4. Signed consent forms (see Chapter 2) have been obtained.

5. A full list of the patients' names, wards, proposed operations and type of anaesthesia (general or local with sedation). Ensure that this list is circulated as soon as possible to all involved wards, the theatre and the anaesthetic department, and that the operating surgeon is informed.
6. Discuss the order of the patients on the list with senior colleagues, preferably the operating surgeon. Generally speaking, young or anxious patients, day cases and diabetic patients should be first on the list. Major or lengthy cases and trauma cases are often placed at the end of a list.
7. Inform the theatre supervisor of any special requirements such as a plating set, special instruments or handpieces such as oscillating saws.

EMERGENCY SURGERY

When emergency or out-of-hours theatre lists are required, the following steps should be taken:

1. Establish a working diagnosis and the degree of urgency for surgery – e.g. respiratory embarrassment and severe haemorrhage require urgent attention.
2. Ascertain when the patient last had anything to eat or drink.
3. Contact the surgeon and find out the preferred time for operation. With multitrauma patients try and fit in with the operating schedule of the parent surgical unit to avoid the patient making several visits to the operating theatre.
4. Obtain written consent if possible.
5. Contact the theatre, inform them of the patient, the name of the operating surgeon and the proposed operation, and try to fix a theatre time.
6. Advise the anaesthetist who will premedicate the patient, and the ward who will prepare the patient for theatre.
7. If plans change or there are delays, then inform theatre, surgeon, anaesthetist and ward in that order. Ask the ward to relay the reasons for changes or delay to the patient.

The operating theatre

Strict discipline is essential in the operating theatre to ensure a clean operating environment and minimal time-wasting.

THEATRE PROCEDURES

For the house officer, attending the operating theatre can be either a thoroughly enjoyable experience when things go smoothly, or a nightmare when things do not go according to plan. To ensure that things do go smoothly, the house officer must:

1. Be early and ensure that the patient has been called for.
2. Check the notes to confirm the planned surgery and the site and side of the operation.
3. Display all the relevant radiographs and models.

4. Ensure all special instruments (plating or implant kit), prosthetic devices (plates or dental implants) and other extraordinary materials (amalgam for apicectomies, synthetic bone grafts, etc.) are available and ready for use.

5. Be generally helpful when not assisting by standing well away from the surgical field and personnel who are scrubbed, calling for the next case, adjusting the operating lights and conveying messages to and from the operating team.

SCRUBBING

Before commencing, make sure all last-minute tasks (e.g. shaving the operative area) are completed and that your safety glasses and face-mask are adjusted to your satisfaction.

1. Adjust the water temperature and outlet pressure of the tap as required.
2. Note the time when scrubbing is commenced.
3. Begin by washing hands and arms with soap two or three times, rinsing under running water each time and draining from the elbows into the basin and not on the floor (2–3 minutes).
4. The next step is to use the surgical scrubbing solution (providone-iodine or chlorhexidine), lathering fingers, hands and arms progressively up to the elbows; do this two or three times, thoroughly rinsing under the tap each time (2–3 minutes).
5. Use of a sterile brush should be confined to scrubbing the fingernails, since scrubbing the skin with a brush tends to expose the deeper microflora of the skin, quite apart from the skin damage vigorous brushing may do (2–3 minutes).
6. At the completion of the scrub, turn off the tap with your elbows and keep your hands facing upwards to allow all free water to drain from the elbows into the scrub sink.
7. Move carefully to the gowning area, ensuring you do not touch anything and keeping your hands facing upwards. Avoid standing behind people and keep well away from the gowning area until it is clear for you to move close.
8. Pick up a sterile towel and dry one hand at a time first and then one arm at a time last.

GOWNING AND GLOVING

1. Pick up the gown which is folded inside out and hold it from the inside by the shoulders (Figure 17.3).
2. Shake the gown, which will unfold, and begin dressing by placing one arm at a time into each of the sleeves while an assistant ties you up at the back.
3. Without touching the outer glove surface, place the right hand into the right glove holding the inner surface of the folded rim with the left hand (Figure 17.4).

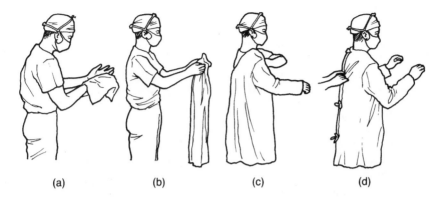

Figure 17.3 Gowning procedure: a, dry hands thoroughly with sterile towel; b, unfold the gown and hold it only from the inside; c, place arms into sleeves one at a time; d, scout nurse (unscrubbed) should tie the back of the gown (after Howe).

4. Place the left hand into the left glove by holding the cuffed outer surface of the glove with the gloved right hand.
5. With both gloves on, evert the cuffs of the gloves to cover the cuffs of the gown sleeves.
6. Fasten the waist tie by asking a scrubbed colleague to hold the tie as you twist to your left then tie it to your waist. This manoeuvre will cover the unsterile back of your gown.
7. Stand back and observe the 'no touch technique'. Sterility is now only ensured from 'nipple to navel', so keep your inactive hands within the confines of this area.

DRAPING

Draping the patient is done to isolate the operative field.

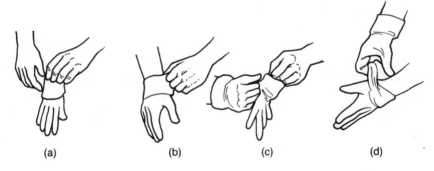

Figure 17.4 Gloving technique. Once the gown is on, gloving can commence: a, pick up the first glove at the rolled cuff; b, insert one hand into the correct glove (labelled left or right) as the other hand steadies the glove then draws it back over the cuff of the gown; c, with the gloved hand, pick up the second glove from under the cuff and bring it up to the other hand; d, bring the cuff of the glove over the sleeve cuff of the gown. *Note:* you are now sterile from 'nipple to navel' so keep your hands within these boundaries.

1. Make sure that the endotracheal tube is adequately secured, the patient's eyes are closed and protected with a light dressing, and a proper head position and support are established.
2. Prepare the operative field with an aqueous-based antiseptic solution, which should be applied in concentric circles, then dried and the procedure repeated two or three times using a sterile gauze for each manoeuvre. Hand the preparation tray and solution to the circulating nurse when finished.
3. Always place the body drape first, preferably in two layers, and include a plastic sheet over the chest.
4. For minor oral surgery procedures, a split drape that exposes the mouth may be sufficient.
5. For more major surgical procedures, a turban head drape is used and the endotracheal tube is covered with a transparent adhesive plastic drape. In some centres, the whole face is covered with an adhesive plastic drape and a small hole is cut to provide access to the operative field.
6. Bring the table up to the operating position and help the nurse set up the suction, drills and diathermy required for surgery.

ASSISTING THE SURGEON

The main objective of assisting is to provide the surgeon with unimpeded access to the operative field at all times.

1. *Retraction* – the assistant must stand in a position where the operative field can be seen (not always possible) and the retractors are held in a comfortable manner that will minimize fatigue. The positioning of the retractors is at the total discretion of the operating surgeon so the assistant must relax the grip on the retractor when the surgeon is attempting to reposition it.
2. *Suction* – keeping the field clear of blood and irrigation solution requires a sensible approach that does not interfere with the surgeon's line of sight or instrumentation. It is best to place the suction at the most gravitationally dependent point in the operative field, preferably on bone.
3. Be alert to anticipate the surgeon's next move and any difficulties encountered. Feed instruments and swabs back to the nurse as necessary.
4. Ask if you become concerned about the patient's colour, handpiece or diathermy function, or some endangered vital structure.
5. Ensure that you can see well enough when cutting sutures as directed.
6. Do not hesitate to warn the surgeon if you are not feeling well and need to unscrub.

END OF OPERATION

Upon completion of the operation the house officer is expected to perform the following duties:

● **Write up the operation record** – which must include the names of the surgeon, assistants and anaesthetist, date of operation and operative diagnosis. In clear and legible handwriting, the title of the surgery and details of the operation should be recorded in an orderly and succinct style under the following headings (Figure 17.5):

   title of operation (e.g. removal of four wisdom teeth)

   incisions and type of flaps used

   dissection carried out, bone removal and/or teeth divided

   teeth or pathological material removed. Biopsy specimens procured for diagnosis

   other abnormal findings

   intraoperative difficulties encountered (e.g. severe haemorrhage)

   wound closure, sutures used and any packs or drains left in situ

   any topical medicaments applied (e.g. haemostatic agents) or infiltrations of local anaesthetic solution into wound.

   The operation sheet must then be signed. If in doubt about certain aspects of the operation, ask the operating surgeon for assistance.

- **Written instructions for postoperative care** – should include notes on:

   when the oral haemostatic packs can be removed

   when the patient can begin oral intake

   the type of diet (liquid or soft)

   wound care, e.g. oral hygiene measures

   patient handling and positioning, e.g. avoid pressure on elevated zygoma so patient to be placed for recovery on the opposite side face down, or instructions to raise the head on several pillows when sleeping and prevent the patient sleeping on operated side of the face

   regular eye observations, particularly where zygomatico-orbital surgery is performed

   contact names and numbers in event of queries or emergency.

- **Postoperative medications** – the patient's drug chart for the ward should be filled out with consideration given to the following medication:

   patient's own regular medication, e.g. salbutamol inhaler, antihypertensive medication, etc.

   analgesics, e.g. parenteral narcotics or oral NSAID/narcotic combinations (see Chapter 13)

   antiemetics, e.g. 10 mg metoclopramide IM six-hourly prn, especially where narcotics are prescribed

   antibiotics (IV or oral) – optional for minor oral surgery (see Chapter 8)

   sleeping aids, e.g. temazepam 10–30 mg orally at night as required, since many patients find it difficult to sleep in the strange hospital environment

   antacids – may be useful for patients stressed by major surgery or trauma

   steroids – commenced in theatre and continued postoperatively to help minimize swelling after major surgery (see Chapter 13).

- **Intravenous fluid orders** (see below) – most important in major surgery where oral intake may be compromised for a few days. For minor oral surgery the litre of Hartmann's solution given at the start of the operation may be all the intravenous fluid required, unless the patient is vomiting, in which case intravenous fluids should continue until vomiting ceases (see Chapter 13).

OPERATION RECORD   **DISTRICT GENERAL HOSPITAL**

PATIENT...... *John Barry Smithson* .... HOSP NO............. *321000* ....

DEPARTMENT..... *Oral & Maxillofacial Surgery* ....

CONSULTANT SURGEON..... *George Dimitroulis* ....

CONSULTANT ANAESTHETIST..... *Gordon Smith* ....

ASSISTANT(S)..... *John Sheen (Senior House Officer)* ....

DIAGNOSIS...... *Impacted Teeth* ....

OPERATION..... *Surgical extraction of 18,28,38,48.* ....

DATE OF OPERATION ...... *14   5 / 96* ...   DURATION..... *35 mins* ......

DETAILS OF OPERATION:

   18 and 28 - Simple elevation

   38 - Surgical removal
       - buccal flap raised
       - buccal bone removed with round bur
       - tooth elevated intact
       - wound toilet
       - closure with 3 x 3/0 chromic catgut sutures

   48 - Surgical removal
       - buccal flap raised
       - buccal bone removed with round bur
       - tooth divided vertically and elevated in 2 pieces
       - wound toilet
       - closure with 3 x 3/0 chromic catgut sutures

             8mls 0.5% marcaine infiltrated

POST-OPERATIVE ORDERS:

1. Routine post-operative care and post-anaesthetic observation
2. Remove oral packs 20 mins after patient enters recovery area
3. Strong light and suction by bedside at all times
4. Replace fresh oral packs if persistent bleeding
5. Nil orally until fully conscious, thereafter soft diet
6. Begin gentle chlorhexidine mouthwashes 8 hrs after surgery

---

SIGNATURE...

PRINT NAME..... *John Sheen (SHO)* ....

CONTACT NO..... *Bleeper - 654321* ....

Figure 17.5 Example of operation notes. One of the most essential items to include is the contact or pager number of the surgeon in case of queries or emergency.

Ward duties

POSTOPERATIVE CARE OF INPATIENTS

Postoperative care is simple in healthy patients who have undergone minor oral surgery, but becomes complex after major surgery and in medically compromised patients.

- Examination of the surgical wound (including donor site) – the wound must be inspected daily while patient remains in hospital. Check for significant pain, bleeding, discharge or wound dehiscence.
- Dressings – are often removed 24–48 hours after surgery. They are replaced with non-adhesive dressings only if there is an open wound or copious discharge, or if the wound is constantly irritated by clothing.
- Drain tubes – check amount of drainage in the previous 24 hours. Make sure vacuum drains are still functioning. Remove drains when there is little or no drainage (usually 1–3 days). Drains kept in too long can result in ascending infection.
- Suture removal – for extraoral wounds (e.g. coronal incision, chest flap, etc.) may be undertaken on a progressive basis, e.g. every second stitch or staple may be removed on day 5–7 and the rest of the sutures or staples removed at 10 days.

ROUTINE WARD DUTIES

Patient progress reports
Patients admitted to the ward for oral and maxillofacial surgery should be visited by the house officer at least twice daily. The patient's progress in terms of surgical wound healing and general physical and mental well-being must be carefully monitored and recorded in the progress notes of the patient's history.

Intravenous fluid therapy
Intravenous fluid administration should be evaluated daily with the objective of stopping IV fluids as soon as the patient is able to take adequate amounts of fluids by mouth. It is recommended that the IV access is changed every 2–3 days to minimize the risk of infection and phlebitis. Healthy adults require 3 litres of fluid daily, e.g. 1 litre each of 5% dextrose, normal saline and Hartmann's solution. Patients with cardiac or renal disease may require less, and those with vomiting, diarrhoea, wound drainage and fever require more. The hydration status of the patient may be monitored with daily urea and electrolyte tests or, in intensive care units, using a central venous pressure line and urinary catheters. If fluid overload occurs, sit the patient upright, slow the infusion and give a diuretic such as 40 mg frusemide.

Medication
Ensure that there are clear instructions to nursing staff about when to stop parenteral administration of drugs and to commence oral intake. Most hospital drug charts require exact times of the day when the drugs should be administered, e.g. 0800, 1600, 2400, rather than simply every 8 hours.

Practical procedures
Every house officer must be familiar with certain routine procedures which require simple instruction and plenty of practice to master. Begin by finding an experienced colleague who can demonstrate and supervise your first attempts. From then on it is 'practice makes perfect'. These procedures include:

blood pressure measurements
venepuncture – for collection of blood samples (Figure 17.6)
intravenous infusion
arterial blood gas measurements
intramuscular and subcutaneous injections
catheterization of the urinary tract
nasogastric intubation
endotracheal intubation (the best place to practice is in theatre under the guidance of the anaesthetist)

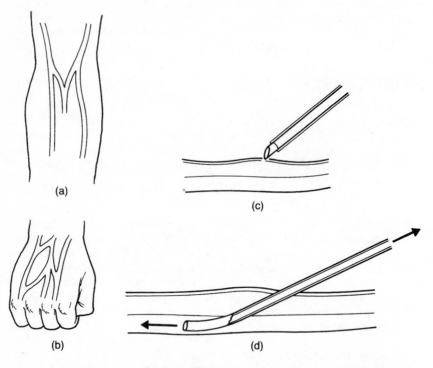

Figure 17.6 Venepuncture technique: a, the antecubital fossa of the arm often has a good selection of large veins that are readily visible for venepuncture (this site is more often used for drawing blood samples than for inserting intravenous catheters); b, the dorsal plexus of veins on the non-dominant hand is the preferred site for intravenous catheters, imparting greater comfort and mobility to patients; c, intravenous catheters are inserted at a 30° angle to the surface of the skin with the bevel of the needle facing down; d, once the vein is penetrated and there is a 'flashback' of blood seen within the chamber of the catheter, the sheath is advanced into the lumen of the vein as the needle is momentarily stabilized, then gradually withdrawn from the catheter.

insertion of a chest drain
application of ECG electrodes.

Tracking results
It is the responsibility of the house officer to maintain an updated record of each patient's haematology, biochemistry, microbiology, pathology and radiology results. There is no excuse for waiting until written reports are sent to the ward. Each request for investigations must be followed up by telephone calls to the relevant departments. Computer technology allows most results to be obtained through the terminals on each ward. When a senior colleague queries an investigation, the house officer must be ready with the most up-to-date results.

Liaison with other specialties
The major advantage of working in a large hospital is the access to a wide range of medical and paramedical specialties available within a single institution. Therefore, when the advice or services of a specialist such as a cardiologist, physiotherapist, dietary expert or social worker are required, it is a matter of a simple telephone call, followed up by a short interdepartmental referral note in the patient's record. In this way total patient care is made possible within a single admission. It is always helpful to know colleagues from other specialties and departments on a social basis, so that when the time comes for requesting their assistance, the response will be prompt and much more productive.

Ward rounds
Ward rounds are essential daily activities that provide a means of updating the status of the patients on the ward, and are particularly important for house officers and students as a teaching exercise in total patient care.

1. Ward rounds should be conducted at least once a day, preferably first thing in the morning.
2. Arrive early and make sure you are totally familiar with the case details for each of the patients on the ward, and take particular note of any new admissions over the preceding 24 hours.
3. Have all radiographs and updated results available for perusal by senior colleagues.
4. Inform the charge sister of the ward when the round will be commencing so that a representative of the nursing staff can be present to take notes on clinical decisions made during the round.
5. Before commencing the ward round, brief senior colleagues of any major, urgent or confidential problems before entering the ward.
6. Lead the ward round to each patient's bedside and present a concise clinical summary with brief mention of the important results of any procedures and relevant investigations. Avoid raising contentious issues within earshot of the patient.
7. Keep an eye on the patient during the round in case comments have been misconstrued, and if so, return to the patient's bedside at the end of the ward round to clarify.

8. Keep notes during the round so that at the end you can record in the patient's notes what future management has been decided.

Discharging patients

1. Give the ward and the patient at least 12 hours notice of intention to discharge.
2. Make sure the patient has a place to return to and family or friends to provide care. If not, contact the social workers who will handle the necessary arrangements for accommodation and care.
3. The patient must be provided with all the necessary discharge medications and clear instructions on how to take them, including written dietary advice, and what to do and whom to contact in event of an emergency.
4. A postoperative outpatient review appointment must be arranged prior to discharge and the patient provided with a written record of the appointment.
5. A letter detailing the patient's hospital stay should be dictated and sent to the patient's own physician and dentist, preferably within 7 days of the discharge date.

POSTOPERATIVE PROBLEMS

During postoperative recovery, on the ward, patients may experience one or more of the following complications, which require prompt attention from the house officer (see also Chapters 13 and 16).

Hypotension

During their hospital stay, all patients normally have vital signs such as blood pressure monitored on a regular basis. Where the blood pressure falls below 100/60 mmHg, it is prudent to investigate the cause and treat accordingly. If the cause is pain, then provide adequate analgesia. More often it is due to inadequate hydration of the patient, requiring intravenous infusion of fluids (especially colloids) to restore circulatory volume and hence pressure. Consider also the possibility of drug overdose (especially narcotics) which may be reversed in emergency cases using naloxone.

Haemorrhage

Minor haemorrhage may be managed in the ward as outlined in Chapter 14. Major haemorrhage will require colloidal, plasma and blood replacement to be commenced immediately in the ward until an emergency operating theatre, surgeon and anaesthetist can be arranged to manage the bleeding. In some cases interventional radiologists may be called upon to track the bleeding source and plug the leak with transcatheter arterial embolization.

Wound infection and breakdown

Inspect the wound daily and keep it clean with daily changes of dressings. Send specimens of wound exudate for microbiological culture and sensitivity tests. For major wound breakdown return to the patient theatre for surgical debridement with open packing of the wound (if not on the face). Antibiotics should be considered.

Deep venous thrombosis and pulmonary embolism
Unless the patient has had surgery in the pelvis or leg for harvesting grafts, or major flap reconstruction, there is little reason why patients who have undergone oral and maxillofacial surgery cannot be ambulatory within 24–48 hours after their operation. Early ambulation helps minimize the incidence of deep venous thrombosis (DVT) and the risk of pulmonary emboli (PE). Furthermore, patients at risk of DVT undergoing lengthy oral and maxillofacial surgery should be fitted with compression stockings, provided with intermittent calf stimulation during surgery and considered for low-dose prophylactic heparin (5000 units given subcutaneously every 8 hours). Oral contraception should be stopped at least 1 month prior to major elective maxillofacial surgery.

Fever
A persistent rise in body temperature greater than 1 °C occurring more than 48–72 hours after surgery is cause for concern and should be investigated.

- **Possible causes** – include local surgical wound infection, distant infection arising from an IV or urinary catheter, allergic response to medication or even a myocardial infarct.
- **Investigations:**
    full blood examination
    chest X-ray
    specimens of wound exudate, sputum, urine and blood for microbiological staining and culture
    ECG and liver function tests.
- **Management** – depends on cause:
    symptomatic – external body cooling, NSAIDs
    local measures – drain pus or haematoma, remove necrotic tissues or foreign bodies, remove infected IV cannulas and catheters
    systemic measures – antibiotics, medical treatment of myocardial infarction or thyroid crisis, surgical treatment of pulmonary embolus.

Cardiorespiratory arrest
If you happen to be in the vicinity when this occurs, call for help and immediately assess airway, breathing and circulation. Commence cardiopulmonary resuscitation (see Chapter 16) until the emergency 'crash team' arrives – they will immediately take over, so stand back and keep out of their way.

Outpatient clinics

PATIENT FOLLOW-UP

When patients are discharged from hospital, review appointments are made for them to be seen in outpatient clinics. These clinics are often fully booked and sometimes overbooked, leaving little time for the patients to be seen by senior colleagues. Therefore the house officer is required to see the backlog of patients, remove splints and wires, chase results, fill out the surgical waiting-list cards, arrange referrals to other departments and keep track of continuing patient care.

REFERRAL OF MEDICALLY COMPROMISED PATIENTS FOR MINOR ORAL SURGERY

Other specialist units will refer their patients for assessment and management. These patients may be referred for dental extractions or other minor oral surgery procedures that are vital to their overall health and well-being. Such patients may include the following:

- Patients who have had open heart surgery or are being considered for open heart surgery.
- Patients who have had organ transplant surgery or are being considered for organ transplantation, in particular heart, heart–lung or liver transplants.
- Patients with chronic renal failure – renal dialysis or renal transplant.
- Patients with acute blood dyscrasias – e.g. leukaemia.
- Cancer patients treated by radiotherapy or chemotherapy.

Management of these patients entails specific requirements essential to their safety and well-being when undergoing minor oral surgery. Such patients should always be treated within a hospital environment. Generally speaking, oral disease in some of these patients can prove morbid or even fatal, so every step must be taken to ensure that long-term oral health needs are never neglected in any way. The reading list below provides further discussion of this topic.

Further reading

Brown AFT (1990) *Accident and Emergency Diagnosis and Management*. Oxford: Butterworth-Heinemann.

Hope RA, Longmore JM, Hodgetts TJ, Ramrakha PS (1994) *Oxford Handbook of Clinical Medicine*. 3rd edn. Oxford University Press.

Lowry JC (1995) Thromboembolic disease and thromboprohylaxis in oral and maxillofacial surgery: experience and practice. *Br J Oral Maxillofac Surg*, **33**, 101–106.

Poswillo D, Babajews A, Bailey M, Foster M (1986) *Dental Oral and Maxillofacial Surgery: A Guide to Hospital Practice*. London: Heinemann.

Robinson R, Stott R (1989) *Medical Emergencies Diagnosis and Management*. 5th edn. Oxford: Butterworth-Heinemann.

Scully C (1989) *Patient Care – A Dental Surgeon's Guide*. London: British Dental Journal.

Swash M (1989) *Hutchison's Clinical Methods*. 19th edn. London: Baillière Tindall.

Turner R, Blackwood R (1990) *Lecture Notes on History Taking and Examination*. Oxford: Blackwell.

Wagner JD, Moore DL (1991) Preoperative laboratory testing for the oral and maxillofacial surgery patient. *J Oral Maxillofac Surg*, **49**, 177–182.

Ziccardi VB, Saini J, Demas PN, Braun T (1992) Management of the oral and maxillofacial surgery patient with end-stage renal disease. *J Oral Maxillofac Surg*, **50**, 1207–1212.

18 Introduction to maxillofacial surgery

Maxillofacial surgery is an essential service carried out by highly skilled individuals who often go through a protracted course of intensive training in both surgery and dentistry. The aim of this chapter is to outline the principles and scope of maxillofacial surgery which may be of particular interest to those wishing to pursue a career in this exciting and rapidly growing field of surgery.

Terminology

Oral and maxillofacial surgery – a regional specialty or surgery dealing with the diagnosis and management – surgical or otherwise – of diseases, injuries and defects of the human jaws and associated structures.
Oral surgery – an old term that has now been largely superseded by the term defined above, owing to the expanded scope of this field.
Maxillofacial surgery – literally, surgery of the jaws and face. In the context of this chapter, the term is used to describe all the surgical procedures undertaken by oral and maxillofacial surgeons other than minor oral surgery.

Scope of oral and maxillofacial surgery

- **Standard procedures** – areas of surgery that few surgeons outside the specialty of oral and maxillofacial surgery understand or practice:
    dentoalveolar surgery
    orthognathic surgery
    temporomandibular joint surgery
    implantology
    trigeminal nerve repair.
- **Shared procedures** – these procedures are not unique to the specialty of oral and maxillofacial surgery, and in fact overlap considerably with other surgical specialties such as otolaryngology or plastic and reconstructive surgery:
    maxillofacial trauma
    cleft lip and palate surgery

craniofacial surgery
head and neck surgery
reconstructive surgery
facial aesthetic surgery.

Maxillofacial trauma

Maxillofacial traumatology is the area of surgery dealing with the diagnosis and surgical management of injuries involving the jaws, facial skeleton and associated structures from the frontal bone to the mandible.

Historical background

Although in the first half of the twentieth century the management of maxillofacial injuries was traditionally undertaken by plastic surgeons and ear, nose and throat surgeons, the significance of this area of surgery is that it enabled the first participation of dental surgeons in surgical procedures beyond the confines of the oral cavity. The numerous wars in the twentieth century have tremendously expanded the surgical expertise of the dental surgeon, who often played a pivotal role in the surgical management of facial fractures, particularly where the dental occlusion was involved. As a reflection of this evolutionary period that eventually led to the development of oral and maxillofacial surgery as a dental specialty, maxillofacial trauma today forms the basis of training and is regarded as a stepping stone to other areas of maxillofacial surgery.

Unique features of maxillofacial injuries

Maxillofacial injuries differ from injuries to other parts of the human body in three ways:

risk to airway, which may be directly compromised
presence of teeth, which assists in the alignment and stabilization of fractures
excellent blood supply to the face, which promotes rapid healing.

Aetiology of maxillofacial injuries

In descending order of frequency:

assaults (especially in Western nations)
motor vehicle accidents (in developing nations)
recreational incidents – contact sports
falls – in children, the elderly and epileptic patients
industrial accidents
other – tooth extractions, pathological fractures.

Distribution of maxillofacial injuries

- Most common in adult males aged 18–25 years, from the lower socio-economic classes.
- Alcohol is often a predisposing factor.
- The most common injuries are, in descending order of frequency:
  nasal fractures
  zygomatic fractures
  mandibular fractures – especially condylar fractures
  dentoalveolar fractures.

Note: as a result of the introduction of compulsory seat belt laws in many countries in recent decades, severe middle third facial injuries have fortunately become uncommon.

Principles of management of facial fractures

- **Debridement** – meticulous cleaning of fracture site.
- **Reduction** – alignment of the fractured bone ends.
- **Fixation** – stabilization of the fractured bone; often done nowadays with miniature bone plates and screws (rigid internal fixation).
- **Immobilization** – of fractured jaws in particular – is achieved by wiring the jaws together for 4–6 weeks (intermaxillary wire fixation). With the widespread use of rigid internal fixation, however, use of this procedure is rapidly declining.
- **Functional rehabilitation** – to ensure that function is fully restored to the traumatized region, e.g. prosthetic replacement of teeth lost as a result of the injury.

Orthognathic surgery

Orthognathic surgery refers to the surgical alignment of the jaws in order to achieve a functional skeletal base occlusal relationship and optimum soft tissue balance of the lower half of the face, i.e. nose, lips and chin.

Historical background

Although there have been scattered reports of orthognathic surgical procedures published as far back as the nineteenth century, it was not until the 1960s that the field of orthognathic surgery really developed, with the publication of the first textbook devoted to the subject. The stage was set for the rapid spread of new techniques and ideas about the clinical application of orthognathic surgery for the treatment of various dentofacial deformities that in the past were routinely managed with orthodontics alone. Orthognathic surgery today forms an integral part of most oral and maxillofacial surgery practices, as virtually no other surgeon without dental training practises in this very complex field of surgery. Orthognathic surgery represents one of the few areas of clinical practice that is totally unique to the specialty of oral and maxillofacial surgery.

Goals of orthognathic surgery

Whereas orthodontics is used to correct the position of the teeth relative to the dental arch, orthognathic surgery aims to correct the position of the jaws relative to the cranial base. It is uncommon to perform orthognathic surgery without concomitant orthodontic treatment, as the surgical movements of the jaws relies to a great extent on the alignment and position of the teeth. The most important role for orthognathic surgery lies in the management of malocclusions which harbour a gross jaw discrepancy between the mandible and maxilla. Hence the dentofacial deformity which orthognathic surgery aims to correct is often described in terms of jaw size and position as opposed to simply a dental malocclusion. For example, a class III dentofacial deformity may be the result of a hypoplastic maxilla and a normal sized mandible, a prognathic mandible and a normal maxilla, or even a combination of a prognathic mandible and a hypoplastic maxilla.

Orthognathic surgical techniques

MAXILLARY SURGERY

The maxillae may be moved as a whole or in segments in any combination of horizontal and vertical directions. This is achieved through a Le Fort I maxillary osteotomy, approached by a circumvestibular incision in the labial sulcus that stretches from the maxillary first molar on one side to the first molar on the other side of the maxilla. Terminology often used to describe the movement of the maxillae is as follows:

- **Vertical movements:**
    superior repositioning – *impaction*
    inferior repositioning – *downgraft.*
- **Horizontal movements:**
    anterior repositioning – *advancement*
    increase in transverse dimension of maxilla – *expansion.*

MANDIBULAR SURGERY

The most commonly performed technique used to move the mandible is the sagittal split ramus osteotomy. With this technique the mandible may be surgically repositioned in the following directions:

- Anterior repositioning – *advancement.*
- Posterior repositioning – *setback.*

TREATMENT PROTOCOLS

Orthognathic techniques may therefore be used to treat the following common jaw conditions:

- Vertical maxillary excess – Le Fort I maxillary impaction.
- Vertical maxillary deficiency – Le Fort I maxillary downgraft.

- Maxillary hypoplasia in the horizontal dimension – Le Fort I maxillary advancement with or without maxillary expansion.
- Mandibular retrognathia – bilateral sagittal split ramus osteotomy (BSSO) with advancement.
- Mandibular prognathism – BSSO with setback.
- Combined jaw abnormalities – two jaw or bimaxillary osteotomies.

Temporomandibular joint surgery

Definitions

- **Temporomandibular disorders (TMD)** – a collective term used to describe a number of related conditions that involve the temporomandibular joints (TMJ), masticatory muscles and associated structures, which may present with facial pain, joint noises, limited jaw function and further non-specific symptoms such as earache, headaches, tinnitus, neck and shoulder pains, etc.
- **Internal derangement (ID)** – although classically this term refers to the abnormal relationship between the disc, condyle and eminence (e.g. disc displacement), in a broader sense it may also be used to describe a localized mechanical fault within the joint that interferes with its smooth action.
- **Osteoarthrosis (OA)** – a non-painful, localized degenerative joint disease. Painful conditions are referred to as osteoarthritis.

Historical background

Surgery of the temporomandibular joint first developed in the nineteenth century as a means of releasing joint ankyloses. However, after a relatively quiet period in the first half of the twentieth century, TMJ surgery gathered momentum in the early 1970s as the concept of disc displacement or internal joint derangement was revived in North America. Since then there has been an explosion in TMJ surgical procedures, including the introduction of the sophisticated technology of small joint arthroscopy. Unfortunately, because of poor understanding of joint pathology and the serious lack of standardized indications for operation, TMJ surgery has become a controversial area of clinical practice.

Indications for TMJ surgery

Only about 5% of all patients being treated for TMD may benefit from surgery.

ABSOLUTE INDICATIONS

Temporomandibular joint surgery has a definite and undisputed role in the management of uncommon disorders such as joint ankylosis, tumours and developmental anomalies of the joint.

RELATIVE INDICATIONS

Unfortunately, the role of TMJ surgery in the management of common disorders such as traumatic injuries, internal derangement and osteo-arthrosis is less clear and often ill-defined. These may be further divided as follows.

General indications

Temporomandibular joint surgery for common conditions should only be considered under the following conditions:

- Where the TMD remains refractory to non-surgical therapy.
- Where the TMJ is the source of the pain and dysfunction, hence:
  pain localized to the TMJ
  pain on functional loading of the TMJ
  pain on movement of the TMJ
  mechanical interferences within the TMJ.

Note: the more localized the symptoms are to the TMJ, the more likely it is that surgery will have a favourable outcome.

Specific indications

The type of surgery warranted is dictated by the specific condition the patient presents with (see below).

Options in TMJ surgery

There are four surgical options available for the management of common joint conditions such as internal derangement, as follows.

ARTHROCENTESIS AND LAVAGE

The simplest and least invasive of these surgical techniques involves flushing Hartmann's solution through the superior joint space via two 20-gauge needles.

- Specific indication – persistent closed lock of acute onset, where the patient is unable to open any further than 30 mm interincisal distance.

ARTHROSCOPY

Use of a miniaturized telescope and camera enables direct visual inspection of a surgically undisturbed superior joint space.

- Specific indications – diagnosis, including biopsy. Also useful for cases of chronic closed lock of the jaw. Although arthroscopy has also been used for treatment of joint hypermobility and advanced degenerative joint disease, the therapeutic effects are yet to be adequately proved.

MODIFIED CONDYLOTOMY

In a modified condylotomy the condylar process is surgically separated from the rest of the mandible, eliminating the need to directly breach the internal joint space.

- Specific indications – used where the patient is able to open more than 40 mm with transient internal joint interferences (i.e. a painful click), but is only pain-free when wearing an occlusal splint, i.e. where there is painful disc displacement with reduction.

ARTHROTOMY

Arthrotomy is a formal open joint procedure where the TMJ is surgically exposed and displayed, usually via a preauricular incision. The most versatile surgical technique of all, it permits a virtually unlimited combination of procedures to be performed.

- Specific indications – particularly useful where there is gross degenerative joint disease and where there is compromised structural integrity of the disc (e.g. perforation).

Note: TMJ surgery *must* always be backed by non-surgical therapy before and after operation, such as occlusal splint therapy and medication.

Implantology

Implantology comprises the technique where alloplastic material is placed into or onto a jaw bone to support a dental prosthesis. Dental implantology is a special area of dentistry that involves two distinct areas of clinical practice – prosthodontics, and oral and maxillofacial surgery.

Historical background

Replacement of missing teeth dates back to the time of the ancient Egyptians; however, it was only after the Second World War that serious attempts were made to anchor prosthetic teeth directly to the jaw bone. Many implant systems were devised, although few stood the test of time.

In the 1970s the first steps were taken to determine the efficacy and safety of the multitude of implant systems that were appearing on the market, through the introduction of a set of specific criteria that were standardized and reproducible so that different implant systems could be compared and objectively scrutinized.

Criteria for implant success

The minimum accepted criterion for a successful implant system is where the dental implant has been shown to provide functional service for 5 years in at least 85% of cases.

THE IDEAL IMPLANT

The ideal dental implant has the following qualities:

biocompatible
adequate mechanical strength to resist masticatory forces
maximum anchoring surface of implant (i.e. maximum surface contact area between implant and bone) requiring minimal bone loss or destruction for fixation purposes
surface microstructure of implant favours healing of bone and gingival tissues.

EVALUATION OF IMPLANT SYSTEMS

- **Objective evaluation:**
  stability (mobility) of implant
  peri-implant bone integrity and health
  peri-implant gingival integrity and health
  major complications – implant fracture, nerve damage, damage to adjacent teeth, violation of maxillary sinus or nasal passages.
- **Subjective evaluation:**
  functional status
  improved aesthetics
  comfort/discomfort
  emotional and psychological attitude of patient to implant.

SUCCESSFUL IMPLANT SYSTEMS

Of all the implant systems available on the market today, most are based on the highly successful Branemark (Nobelpharma) osseointegration screw technique (see below). Another type of successful implant system is the transmandibular implant (TMI) of Bosker.

Osseointegrated endosseous screw implants

OSSEOINTEGRATION

Osseointegration is the direct structural and functional connection between the surface of a loaded implant and living bone which remodels in accordance with the masticatory forces it is subjected to.

COMPONENTS OF THE BRANEMARK (NOBELPHARMA) IMPLANT SYSTEM

- Titanium fixtures – a screw of 3.75 mm diameter and length varying from 7 mm to 20 mm. This is inserted into jaw bone with an atraumatic surgical technique and left to osseointegrate within the bone from 3 months (in mandible) to 6 months (in maxilla) before it is attached to and loaded with a prosthesis.
- Transmucosal abutment cylinder and gold centres screw – These are inserted after the fixture has fully osseointegrated. The cylinder and

screw help to anchor the prosthesis directly to the titanium fixture within the bone.

Transmandibular implant of Bosker

BACKGROUND

The transmandibular implant system was developed by the Dutch in the 1970s to overcome the problem of implant-bearing capacity in severely atrophic mandibles.

COMPONENTS

Made of precious metals, the basic components include a lower border base plate, numerous cortical screws to fix the base plate to the mandible, and numerous transosseous and transmucosal posts that are connected by a dolder bar in the mouth. The lower prosthesis is then attached to the dolder bar which stabilizes it against the normal masticatory forces.

Implant failure

Failure of the implant may arise from :

- The implant system – particularly the newer systems where no long-term data are available for comparison with tried and proven systems.
- The clinician – mainly owing to poor treatment planning or inexperience, resulting in awkward fixture placement in poor locations (e.g. sinus or close to inferior dental nerve) or inadequate alignment/parallelism between fixtures so that the construction of the prosthesis is compromised.
- The patient – usually owing to poor healing secondary to underlying systemic disease (e.g. diabetes) or poor compliance (e.g. poor oral hygiene) and infection.

Other areas of maxillofacial surgery

Since the demand for some areas of maxillofacial surgery is small (with the exception of facial aesthetic surgery), one way to maintain the skills of the few surgeons trained in these areas is to broaden the referral base and centralize the service. In this way the experience and development of a highly specialized surgical unit are continuously nurtured with a constant flow of patients. It is unproductive, for example, to train all oral and maxillofacial surgeons in craniofacial surgery when the need for such a service is strictly limited.

Cleft lip and palate surgery

Cleft lip and palate surgery is a multistaged surgical discipline that deals with the surgical correction of a distinct congenital facial deformity.

Surgery may begin with the primary repair of a cleft lip at 2–3 months of age and continue with numerous surgical procedures well into early adulthood.

Craniofacial surgery

First developed in the 1960s, craniofacial surgery is a highly specialized area of surgery that deals with the surgical correction of complex congenital and acquired deformities of the cranium, orbits, facial skeleton and jaws.

Head and neck surgery

Dealing with surgical pathology in the head and neck region, head and neck surgery has become a well-recognized subspecialty of otolaryngology in many countries. However, in the UK, continental Europe and some countries in the Far East (e.g. Korea), many oral and maxillofacial surgeons are successfully practising in this area as the primary surgeons.

Reconstructive surgery

Reconstructive surgery is the surgical correction of facial deformities resulting from disease, trauma or maldevelopment. Although a major part of plastic surgery, even sophisticated techniques such as microvascular flap reconstruction are being practised by more and more oral and maxillofacial surgeons worldwide.

Facial aesthetic surgery

Often a purely elective field of surgery, facial aesthetic surgery deals with the surgical manipulation of tissues for the purpose of improving the attractive quality of a given facial appearance. Traditionally the domain of plastic surgeons, the practice of facial aesthetic surgery is rapidly spreading to other surgical specialties such as oral and maxillofacial surgery, particularly in the USA, where a lucrative practice can be easily and quickly established in a very large potential market.

Nerve repair

In oral and maxillofacial surgery, this area mainly deals with the surgical repair of traumatic lesions involving the peripheral sensory branches of the trigeminal nerve.

Conclusion

In most countries of the world, oral and maxillofacial surgery has gained the respect and acceptance it deserves in both the medical and dental professions. This has by no means been an easy task, since the respected status of oral and maxillofacial surgery has been the work of many dedicated surgeons who have had to battle against numerous obstacles to nurture and develop the specialty into what it has become today. Oral and maxillofacial surgery is an exciting and rapidly growing specialty that has undergone tremendous changes in both training requirements and scope of practice. In spite of these great changes and the expanded scope of the specialty, the practice of minor oral surgery still constitutes a substantial part of the day-to-day practice of most oral and maxillofacial surgeons worldwide and will continue to do so for many years to come.

Further reading

Bell WH, ed. (1992) *Modern Practice in Orthognathic and Reconstructive Surgery* Vols I–III. Philadelphia: Saunders.

Branemark P-I, Zarb GA, Albrektsson T (1985) *Tissue Integrated Prostheses: Osseointegration in Clinical Dentistry.* Chicago: Quintessence.

Dimitroulis G, Avery BS (1994) *Maxillofacial Injuries: A Synopsis of Basic Principles, Diagnosis and Management.* Oxford: Butterworth-Heinemann.

Dimitroulis G, Dolwick MF, Van Sickels JA (1994) *Orthognathic Surgery: A Synopsis of Basic Principles and Surgical Techniques.* Oxford: Butterworth-Heinemann.

Dolwick MF, Dimitroulis G (1994) Is there a role for temporomandibular joint surgery? *Br J Oral Maxillofac Surg,* **32**, 307–313.

Dolwick MF, Sanders B (1985) *TMJ Internal Derangement and Arthrosis: Surgical Atlas.* St Louis: Mosby.

Fonseca RJ, Davis WH (1995) *Reconstructive Preprosthetic Oral and Maxillofacial Surgery.* 2nd edn. Philadelphia: Saunders.

Kaban LB (1990) *Pediatric Oral and Maxillofacial Surgery.* Philadelphia: Saunders.

Keith DA (1992) *Atlas of Oral and Maxillofacial Surgery.* Philadelphia: Saunders.

McGregor IA, McGregor FM (1986) *Cancer of the Face and Mouth: Pathology and Management for Surgeons.* Edinburgh: Churchill Livingstone.

Moore JR, ed. (1985) *Surgery of the Face and Mouth.* Oxford: Blackwell.

Peterson LJ (1992) *Principles of Oral and Maxillofacial Surgery.* Philadelphia: Lippincott.

Peterson LJ, Ellis III E, Hupp JR, Tucker MR (1993) *Contemporary Oral and Maxillofacial Surgery.* 2nd edn. St Louis: Mosby.

Williams JLI, ed. (1994) *Rowe and Williams Maxillofacial Injuries.* 2nd edn. Edinburgh: Churchill Livingstone.

Index

NB Page references to figures are italic